# contents

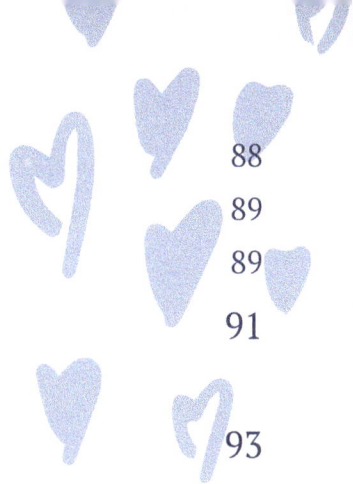

# Pregnancy

## Birth, and Baby Care
## With Essential Oil

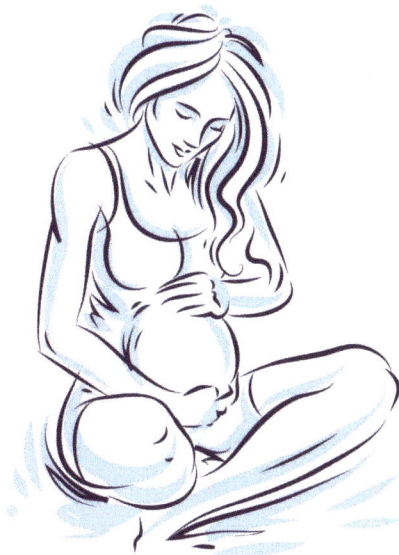

Rebecca Park Totilo

*Pregnancy, Birth, and Baby Care with Essential Oil*

**Disclaimer Notice:** The information contained in this book is intended for educational purposes only and is not meant to substitute for medical care or prescribe treatment for any specific health condition. Please see a qualified healthcare provider for medical treatment. We assume no responsibility or liability for any person or group for any loss, damage, or injury resulting from the use or misuse of any information in this book. No express or implied guarantee is given regarding the effects of using any of the products described herein.

Paperback ISBN:  978-0-9991865-7-2

Electronic ISBN: 978-0-9991865-8-9

# Introduction

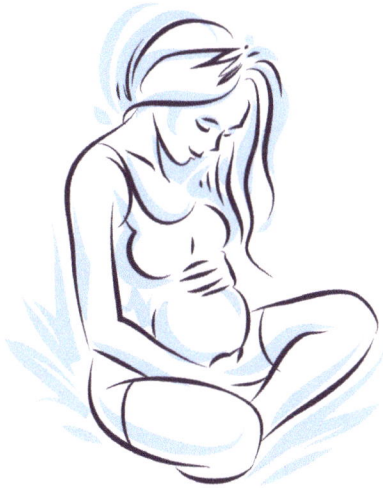

Pregnancy can be an exciting and joyous time in a woman's life, as it highlights her nurturing and creative power to connect the legacy of her past to the future like a string of pearls.

With the joyful anticipation of a new life beginning inside you, utmost care to the health of you and your unborn child must be given when considering aromatherapy as a complementary therapy during pregnancy. A growing body of misinformation and conflicting advice continues to fuel the confusion regarding the use of essential oils during pregnancy. Certain essential oils could cause an adverse effect on the development of your baby (especially in his or her early developmental stages), or cause uterine contractions, leading to a miscarriage. Fortunately, most of these oils are not offered by reputable essential oil companies and can be easily avoided. The majority of essential oils readily available are safe to use during your pregnancy with some exceptions. Those exceptions will be discussed further in detail later as well as the method of application and dosages used during your childbearing year.

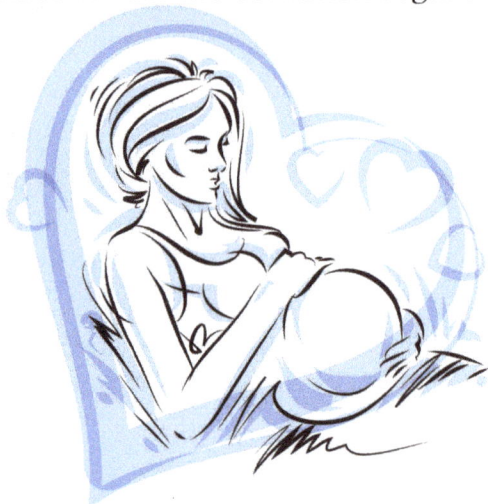

There is a growing body of evidence regarding the benefits of essential oils during pregnancy and birth. It is no wonder so many moms-to-be are looking to a more holistic approach to their prenatal care. From the discomforts of an achy back and swollen feet to sleeplessness and morning sickness, you may find aromatherapy to be a safe form of relief. Here are some of the ways you can benefit from essential oils during your pregnancy:

- Essential oils have a calming effect and relieve stress
- Essential oils can balance your mood and roller-coaster emotions
- Essential oils help with insomnia and nausea
- Essential oils help with body aches and pain
- Essential oils are antiviral, antibacterial, and antiseptic

## Are Essentials Oils Safe to Use During Pregnancy?

While the topic of essential oil usage during pregnancy (especially during the first trimester) is a contentious one, most experts agree that it is highly unlikely using a few drops of essential oil in a warm bath at night will cause any complications or health risks to the unborn child. But, even though there are no recorded cases of miscarriage or birth defects as a result of the normal use of essential oils either topically or by inhalation, myths continue to circulate on the internet that massage oils containing essential oils such as rose or rosemary can cause a miscarriage and should be avoided throughout pregnancy.

Pregnancy Tip: During the first trimester, the use of essential oils should be minimal. This is because of the many changes that are taking place in the mother's body. For this delicate time, it is recommended to refrain from daily use of essential oils unless needed for a specific cause such as morning sickness. By limiting your use, you will still receive the incredible benefits of aromatherapy without overwhelming your senses or overexposing your baby to unnecessary risks.

Battaglia, author of *The Complete Guide to Aromatherapy*, writes, "The judicious use of essential oils together with appropriate forms of massage by a skilled therapist can help ease the discomforts of pregnancy and provide a sense of nurturing that will comfort the mother at times she is likely to be feeling rather fragile." (Battaglia, S. (2002). *The Complete Guide to Aromatherapy*. Australia: International Centre of Holistic Aromatherapy.)

## Are Essential Oils Unsafe for Babies in the Uterus?

No research proves whether or not the inhalation, internal, or topical application of essential oils during pregnancy is a risk factor to the unborn fetus. The book *Aromatherapy for Health Professionals* states, "There's no evidence or even proof that any natural essential oil has ever forced mutagenicity or even teratogenicity in an embryo of a developing fetus. There has never been a test or any carried out because the possibility of fragrant materials is causing either genetic change; this just a malformation which is regarded as unlikely."

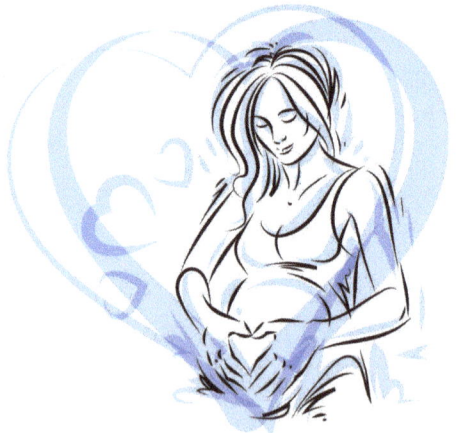

Dr. Jane Buckle, the author of *Clinical Aromatherapy*, writes, "The use of essential oils in pregnancy is a contentious subject, especially during the vital first three-month period. It is improbable that a nightly bath containing a few drops of essential oils will cause any harms for the unborn child." Another word, there are no records of abnormal fetuses or aborted fetuses due to the 'normal' use of essential oils, either by inhalation or topical application."

## Is Aromatherapy Safe During Pregnancy?

The scientific community has failed to provide any compelling evidence that the use of specific essential oils during pregnancy poses any threat or risk to the unborn child. Many women have used essential oils during their pregnancy with no side effects.

Selecting essential oils regarded as safe to use during pregnancy is paramount. With proper dilution and care taken, you will significantly enhance your experience and benefits. Make sure your doctor is aware of your usage of essential oils. Be aware that some oils may have a stimulating effect on the urinary system and uterus and can cross the placental barrier. Also, while nursing a baby, be careful to prevent skin transference to baby and/or through the mother's milk.

## Essential Oils and Pregnancy Risks

One of the main concerns during pregnancy is the risk of essential oil constituents crossing over into the placenta. And, if so, which constituents should we be concerned with? Aromatherapy experts Tisserand and Balacs state that essential oils crossing the placenta does not necessarily mean that there is a risk of toxicity to the fetus; this will depend on the toxicity and the plasma concentration of the compound. (Bensouilah J, and Buck P. *Aromadermatology*. Abingdon, UK: Radcliffe Publishing Ltd.) It is probable that essential oil metabolites cross the placenta due to the intimate (but not direct) contact between maternal and embryonic or fetal blood. (Tisserand, R., and Balacs, T. (1995). *Essential Oil Safety*. New York: Churchill Livingstone.)

## Therapeutic Actions of Essential Oils

In an online article entitled *Pregnancy and Skin Care: Safety Considerations*, author Eve Stahl writes, "Pregnancy is a special time to honor the health of a new life. Proper selection and use of herbs and flowers can enhance the health and strength of mother and fetus. Some plants' functions are considered to be contrary to the optimal support of life during this precious time. It is important to respect the specific functions of each herb (essential oil)."

Stahl states that while some essential oils are emmenagogues, which means their specialized function is to promote and regulate menstruation, they do care for the imbalances of the female reproductive system. The confusion is whether all emmenagogues bring on menstruation and/or are abortifacients and should be avoided during pregnancy. She continues, "Actually, emmenagogues are a class of herbs that function to balance the female reproductive system in a variety of ways. This can be easing pain and cramps during menses, regulating lack of menses, too frequent menses, and excessive mucus during menses. Only some emmenagogue herbs are contraindi-

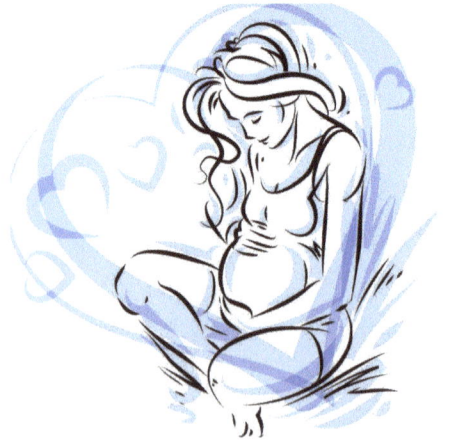

cated during pregnancy." An emmenagogue that serves to relax and ease cramps may not necessarily need to be avoided during pregnancy and will not necessarily prevent conception, cause a miscarriage, or cause other harm.

Besides emmenagogues, another therapeutic property that may alarm you is abortifacient, which means it may induce an abortion. According to world-renowned aromatherapy expert Salvatore Battaglia, he states there is no clear evidence that essential oils are abortifacient. Rather, these essential oils are toxic and are not recommended for use. However, the research referred to in Robert Tisserand's book, *Essential Oil Safety*, indicates oils such as parsley and pennyroyal do have a strong abortifacient action and should be avoided during pregnancy. Other essential oils that are considered abortifacient include mugwort (wormwood), rue, sage, sassafras, savin, thuja, and tansy. For this reason, essential oils should be used with the understanding that they are highly concentrated and readily absorbed by you and your unborn child.

Author Ron Guba points out in an article entitled "Toxicity Myths," that toxicity during pregnancy is almost exclusively due to pregnant women taking large, toxic doses of essential oils, notably pennyroyal (rich in the ketone pulegone, which is metabolized to the highly toxic furan epoxide, menthofuron) and parsley seed (rich in the dimethyl ether apiol) in an attempt to abort the fetus. (Guba, R. (2000). "Toxicity Myths." International Journal of Aromatherapy, Vol. 10.1/2.)

## Do Essential Oils Cross the Placenta?

Because of the low molecular mass of essential oils, there is the potential of the oil crossing the placenta to the fetus. However, this does not mean all essential oils are fetotoxic. It depends on an essential oil's constituents and the plasma concentrations (Tisserand and Balacs, 1999). The concern is that the immature fetal liver would be unable to metabolize the compounds into more toxic ones (unlike adults) thus providing the fetus a degree of protection from any potentially harmful constituents in certain essential oils (Tiran, 2004).

## Which Essential Oils Are Safe During Pregnancy?

Not all essential oils are off-limits during pregnancy. You will find several essential oils that may be helpful during the woes of morning sickness, body aches and pains, edema, and your body's adjustment to pregnancy. Essential oils that are safe during the first trimester include benzoin, bergamot, black pepper, chamomile (Roman and German), coriander, cypress, eucalyptus, fir, frankincense, geranium, ginger, grapefruit, juniper, lavender, lemon, lime, mandarin, marjoram, myrtle, orange, peppermint, petitgrain, rosemary, sandalwood, tangerine, tea tree, and ylang ylang.

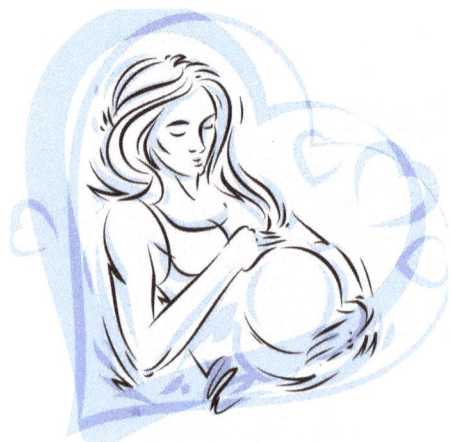

During the second and third trimester, other essential oils are safe for use since your baby is more developed. For instance, you can use certain essential oils that can help with lower back pain and sleeplessness.

Due to the lack of clear information regarding the toxicity of certain oils, the following should be avoided all together: anise star, aniseed, basil, clove bud, fennel, parsley, sage, tarragon, and yarrow. These are all considered phytoestrogens that assist in regulating, stimulating, balancing the body's hormones and enzyme production and may cause contractions. According to Tisserand and Balacs, in addition to this list, other essential oils to avoid include: rue, oakmoss, *Lavandula stoechas*, camphor, and hyssop.

Pregnancy comes with a need for the mother to find the best support of health for her future child. The growing fetus depends entirely on its mother's healthy body for all needs. Consequently, pregnant women must take steps to remain healthy and can add aromatherapy as a part of the many health care and lifestyle considerations. During this special time, by all means, enjoy the wonderful benefits of nature's therapy with essential oils, but do heed caution when using oils during your pregnancy and always use less concentrated formulas than during normal use.

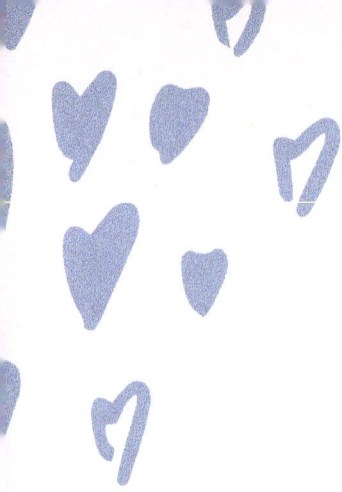

# History Of Aromatherapy

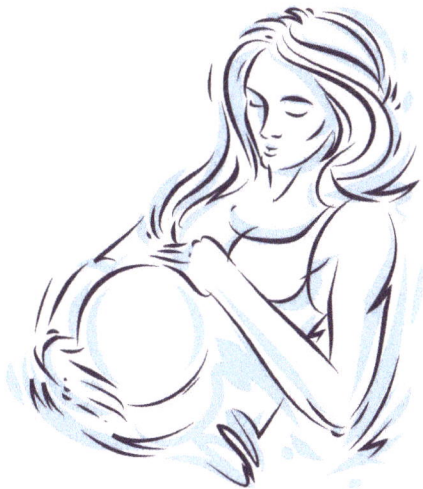

# History of Aromatherapy for Childbirth and Its Benefits During Labor

Undoubtedly, there are very few things in the world that makes a woman more joyful than giving life to another human. For most women, the childbearing experience can be overwhelming, with the fear and dread of labor pain, but in the end, it is very rewarding.

To reduce labor pain, many women have turned to complementary therapies such as aromatherapy, acupuncture, mind-body techniques, and reflexology, among others. Aromatherapy, however, seems to be one of the most effective options for expectant mothers.

## History of Aromatherapy and Childbirth

In 1990, a study was conducted to ascertain the effectiveness of aromatherapy in reducing pain, anxiety, and fear during labor. A total of 8058 mothers in childbirth were subjected to aromatherapy using clary sage and chamomile essential oils. When the study ended in 1997, it was revealed that the use of systemic opioids in the hospital where the study was conducted had decreased from 6% to 0.4%.

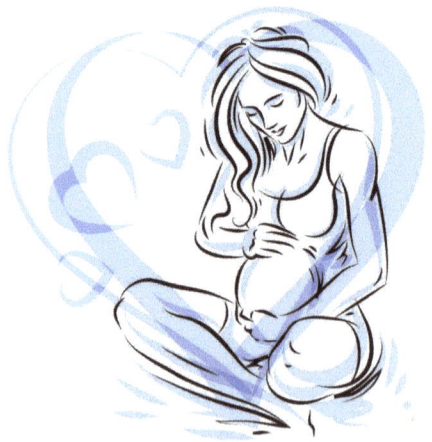

In 2014, another study was conducted, and the findings showed that aromatherapy was effective for alleviating pain intensity and decreasing the duration of labor. The new mothers who were subjected to aromatherapy reported that they were satisfied with the pain relief. The study also revealed that Caesarean sections were reduced significantly. This discovery led to the conclusion that aromatherapy is an affordable nursing intervention that has the potential to reduce pain during labor and improve the labor and delivery experience.

## Benefits of Aromatherapy During Labor

### 1) Helps you relax

Most women become panicky once it's time to give birth to their babies. Naturally, it is to be expected. Unfortunately, anxiety does not make the labor process easier—instead, it can increase your pain and hours in labor. Aromatherapy is known to aid relaxation. It eases tension, calming your mind and body.

### 2) Boosts your mood

A lot of pregnant women have reported that they become irritable and aggressive before and during labor. Aromatherapy can help to improve your mood and keep your emotions in check. It promotes peace of mind and stirs positive emotions. You will need a lot of that during labor.

### 3) Eases physical discomfort, pain, and stress

Aromatherapy decreases cortisol, a stress hormone in the human body. By easing tension and anxiety, the treatment helps to reduce pain perception. It helps expectant mothers feel in control and relaxed. It also helps them to feel supported and nurtured by the midwife or support partner.

### 4) Reduces nausea and vomiting

Aromatherapy is useful for alleviating nausea and vomiting in labor. It makes it easy for women to cope with the discomfort of an upset stomach. Most women experience a heightened sense of smell during pregnancy. Aromatherapy can make the surroundings more comfortable and pleasant during pregnancy and labor.

## 5) Stimulates circulation

Some essential oils are known to stimulate circulation in the body. During pregnancy, your circulatory system works differently. Aromatherapy promotes proper circulation at this time and down into labor. This will increase the wellbeing of you and your new infant.

If you are considering using aromatherapy during your labor to ease pain, you should become familiar with the scent of the essential oil you want to use. Make sure you are comfortable with its aroma before you subject yourself to it during your child's birth.

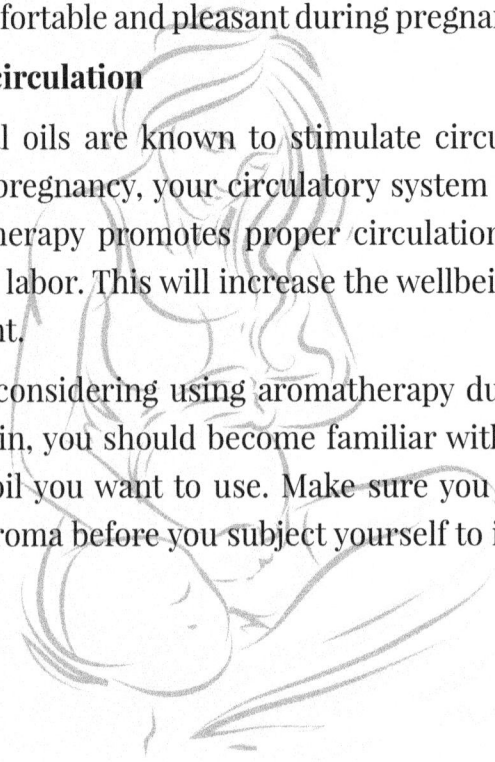

# Aromatherapy Basics

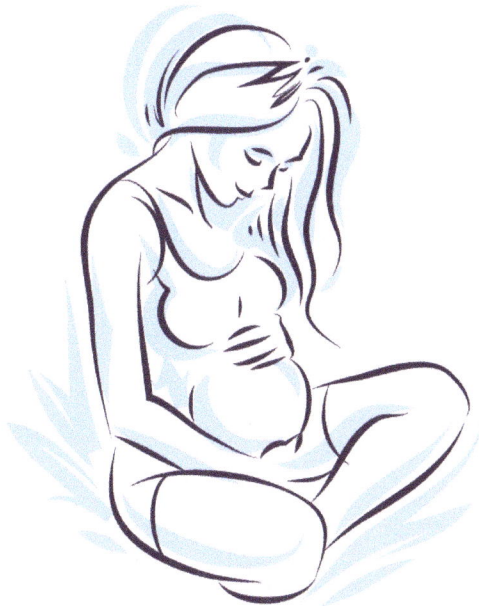

Essential oils are the volatile, aromatic compounds that come from many different parts of plants. They can come from the roots, stems, leaves, flowers, seeds, and other parts of plants. Essential oils in some form have been used since ancient times to support the body through a variety of health, wellness, and beauty concerns. While the essential oils we use today are stronger due to the technology of modern-day distillation practices, the benefits that people experienced in ancient times are still available to us today.

## Distillation

While there are several methods for extracting essential oils, steam distillation and cold-pressing are two of the most common methods. Other popular alternatives to traditional steam distillation include turbo distillation, hydro diffusion and carbon dioxide extraction.

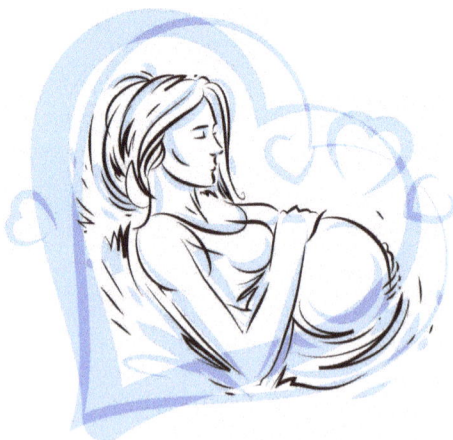

In steam distillation, pressurized steam is sent through the plant material where it bursts opens sacs that contain the essential oils. The essential oils and steam are then sent into a condenser where the steam turns into water, and the essential oil sits on top of the water. The essential oil is then separated from the water and bottled for use. The water contains minute particles of the essential oil and is bottled as hydrosols, another aromatherapy modality.

In cold pressing, the plant material is put under extreme pressure without the use of heat. The pressure breaks open the oil sacs, and the oil is then collected and bottled for use. This type of distillation is mostly used in citrus oils where the rind contains the essential oils.

## Essential Oil Safety

The following are general safety guidelines for using essential oils.

1. Dilute essential oils properly before topical use (see the dilution chart below).

2. Avoid using phototoxic essential oils when you're going to be exposed to the sun. These oils should be used at least 12 hours before sun exposure.

3. Always perform a skin patch test before applying essential oils to a large area of the body.

4. Avoid oxidized oils—store your oils in a cool, dark place in tightly sealed bottles to help ensure they don't oxidize.

5. Keep oils stored where small children and pets cannot get them.

6. Know who you're purchasing your oils from. Check out the GC/MS charts from your suppliers to ensure you're getting the oil you think you're purchasing.

7. Avoid oils that are labeled "for fragrance use only." These are generally synthetics.

8. If you're on medication or dealing with chronic health issues, always consult with a trained aromatherapist before

beginning an aromatherapy treatment.

9. Learn about the oils you're using—look at each oil's safety profile and possible contraindications/reactions before using a new oil.

## Dilution

Dilution is an important part of using essential oils safely and effectively. Dilution decreases the risk of skin sensitivity or adverse reactions when using essential oils topically. Also, when you dilute your oils in a carrier oil, you don't need to use as much essential oil, making it more cost-effective. Paying attention to dilution rates for pregnant women and newborn infants is especially important due to the vulnerability and fragility involved with new life.

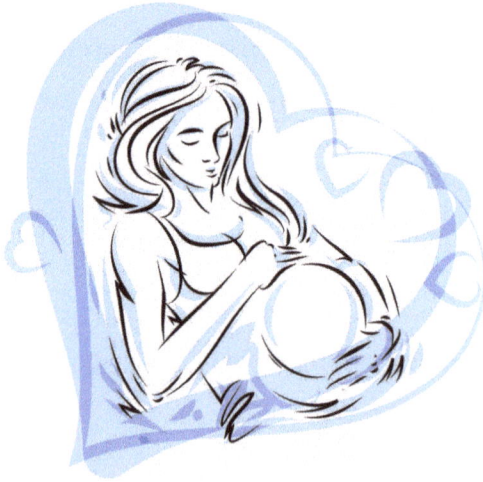

It's always important to use the lowest dilution possible to see if this will give you the results you are seeking. If not, you can add more as needed. Below is a dilution chart that you can use to ensure you're blending safely.

|       | 5 ml | 10 ml | 15 ml | 20 ml | 25 ml | 30 ml | 50 ml | 100 ml |
|-------|------|-------|-------|-------|-------|-------|-------|--------|
| .5%   | .75  | 1.5   | 2.25  | 3     | 3.75  | 4.5   | 7.5   | 15     |
| 1%    | 1.5  | 3     | 4.5   | 6     | 7.5   | 9     | 15    | 30     |
| 2%    | 3    | 6     | 9     | 12    | 15    | 18    | 30    | 60     |
| 3%    | 4.5  | 9     | 13.5  | 18    | 22.5  | 27    | 45    | 90     |
| 4%    | 6    | 12    | 18    | 24    | 30    | 36    | 60    | 120    |
| 5%    | 7.5  | 15    | 22.5  | 30    | 37.5  | 45    | 75    | 150    |

The recommended dilution is 1% for all topical applications (on the skin via massage or compress). In the bath, the mom-to-be should use no more than four drops of essential oil. For lotions or massage oils, use 1-2 drops of essential oil in a teaspoon of carrier oil or lotion. No dilution is needed for diffusion.

## Methods of Delivery

Essential oils can be used in a variety of different ways, including inhalation, topical, and internal. These three methods of application are briefly covered below:

### Inhalation

Inhalation can be accomplished in a variety of ways, including:

- Diffusion
- Personal inhalers
- Adding a few drops to a tissue or cotton ball
- Steam treatments

- Simply opening the bottle and taking a sniff

## *Topical*

Topical use is applying the essential oils directly to the skin's surface. Remember always to use a carrier for topical use. Ways to use essential oils topically include:

- Roller bottle
- Lotion
- Massage oil
- Salve

## *Internal*

During pregnancy and post-partum, the most effective routes of delivery with essential oils when used internally are through rectal supposi-tories or vaginal pessaries. In each of these, the essential oils are generally mixed with a cocoa butter formulation and molded into small, skinny tubes that can easily be inserted into the anus or vagina. The natural heat of the body melts down the cocoa butter and allows the essential oils to be absorbed into the body. This type of use comes in very handy in times of dealing with vaginal yeast infections, constipation, hemorrhoids, vaginal infections, and respiratory illness during pregnancy.

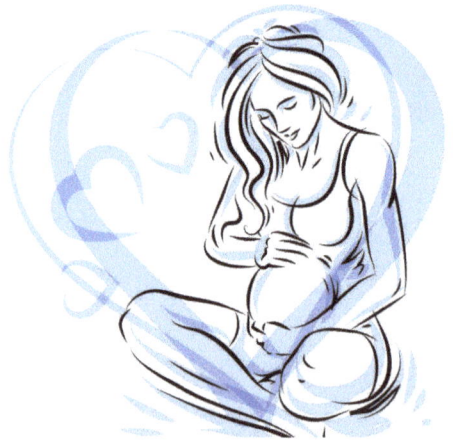

# Best Ways to Use Essentials Oils During Pregnancy

- **Lotions** – Lotions are an excellent method for using essential oils topically. You can purchase an unscented lotion or make your own and add in your essential oils. Lotions work well for muscular pain, digestive issues, and breast care.

- **Creams** – Creams can be used in much the same way lotions are. The main difference is they are thicker. Creams, in pregnancy, can help mom combat any skin dryness or irritation quite nicely.

- **Inhalers** – Inhalers are a mom-to-be's favorite way of using essential oils aromatically. They are simple, portable, and can be used discreetly anywhere. Inhalers are great for fatigue, anxiety, depression, nausea, and vomiting.

- **Roller Bottles** – Roller bottles are a convenient way of using essential oils topically. You can use single essential oils or blends, diluted in carrier oils, that are ready for use when needed. These are great for busy moms, especially when you are out and about.

- **Sitz Baths** – Sitz baths are an effective way of treating hemorrhoids, yeast infections, and Group B Strep. It's important to use only gentle essential oils, diluted properly when using oils on delicate tissue such as the vagina.

- **Compresses** – Compresses are a great way to treat muscular cramps, skin issues, injury, and pain. Compresses can be either cool or warm.

- **Massages** – Touch modalities, such as massage, can go a long way in helping relieve stress, muscle aches, and tension while providing pain relief. In a pregnancy massage, it's important never to rub over the uterus or the breasts. Back or leg massages are fine, provided the mother-to-be is sitting up or laying on her side. Never position a pregnant woman on her stomach for massage work, and if anything causes pain or discomfort immediately stop.

# Tools of the Trade

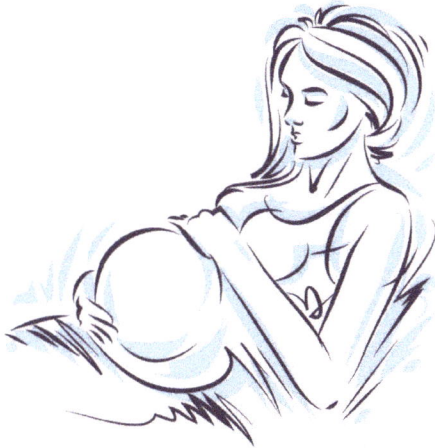

Essential oils are versatile and effective in treating common ailments for pregnancy, labor, and beyond. Their ability to assist in healing physical complaints and postpartum emotional upsets are astounding. You will want to have the necessary equipment available such as bottles, droppers, and containers before starting your aromatherapy blend. Below is a list of the necessary tools you will need to get started:

**Diffusers** – Used to put microscopic droplets of essential oils into the air for aromatic use. While the designs of essential oil diffusers are endless, they generally either require a bottle of essential oil to be attached to a nebulizer itself or drops of essential oils added to the water in the diffuser.

**Roller Bottles** – These are glass bottles that have a roller top on them that are great for using essential oils topically. You can dilute your essential oil or blend with the carrier oil of your choice and have it ready for use when using these bottles.

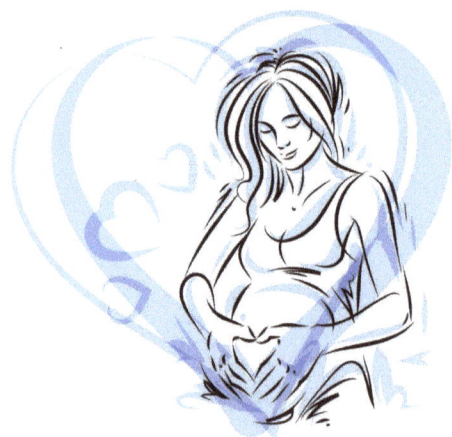

**Dark Glass Bottles** – These are useful for storing essential oils or blends in 5 ml, 15 ml, or 30 ml sizes. The dark glass helps keep the oil from being exposed to light. These are great for storing your essential oil blends.

**Glass Bowls** – Used for mixing ingredients in blending projects or soaking wicks from personal inhalers. These can be purchased online in various sizes.

**Stir Rods** – Rods are convenient for stirring essential oil blends and ingredients together. You can purchase these in glass, stainless steel, or wooden form. However, the wooden ones are for single-use while the glass and stainless steel can be washed and reused.

**Inhalers** – When diffusing is not an option, making personal inhalation blends for use when out and about is the way to go. These come in 4 parts: the cap, the base, the wick, and a small end cap that snaps on the bottom. To use, simply apply your essential oils directly to the wick and assemble the inhaler. Alternatively, you can mix your essential oils in a glass bowl and add the wick to the bowl to absorb the oils, then drop into the canister using tweezers.

**Glass Measuring Cups** – Useful in measuring out ingredients for blending projects. These can also be used as a makeshift double boiler.

**Double Boiler** – This is a small glass or stainless-steel pan insert for melting butter and waxes when making essential oil blending products. These keep the ingredients from being directly heated on the stove or hot plate to keep the ingredients stable.

**Perfume Strips** – Small strips of absorbent paper used to experience the scents of essential oils. These are a great way to introduce your friends or family members to the scents of essential oils they could benefit from as well as seeing how oils may blend together.

**Tweezers** – These will be used to pick up cotton wicks used inside inhalers after absorbing the essential oil and replacing it inside the tube.

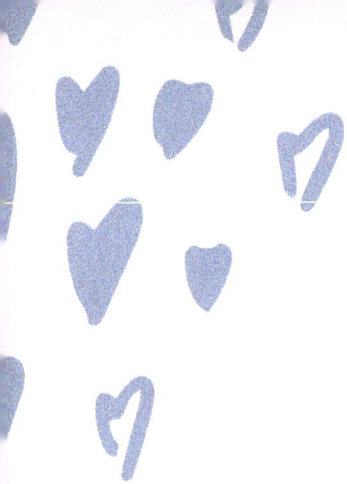

# Essential Oils for Pregnancy

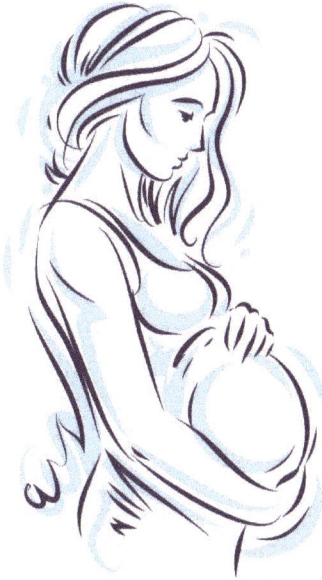

myris (*Amyris balsamifera*) is valued for its refreshing fragrance known to take away stress and anxiety. Because of its delicate aroma, it is a favorite oil in perfume as a fixative, extending the life of the perfume. It is very grounding and soothing to jittery nerves. Amyris essential oil is recommended for helping with falling asleep, as well as improving the appearance of mature skin. This pale yellow oil comes from a tree grown in Haiti and other islands in the Caribbean.

- **Chemical Families:** Alcohols 78%, Sesquiterpenes 12%, Ethers 2%, and Other 8%.

- **Therapeutic Properties:** Anti-anxiety, antiseptic, calming, cicatrizant, and sedative.

- **Safety Data:** There are no known safety concerns with amyris essential oil.

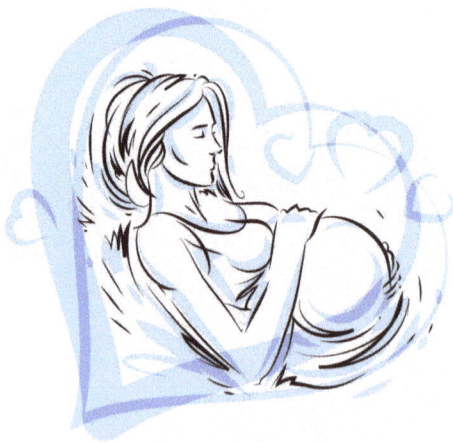

**Balsam Fir** is considered stimulating and can be used to combat the symptoms of colds, cough, flu, and chest congestion with its potent antimicrobial properties. It is also an analgesic and has anti-inflammatory properties, which helps alleviate arthritis and muscular aches and pains.

- **Chemical Families:** Monoterpenes 83%, Esters 13%, Sesquiterpenes 1%, and Other 3%.

- **Therapeutic Properties:** Analgesic, anti-inflammato-

ry, antiseptic, antirheumatic, antispasmodic, decongestant, drying, rubefacient, and is immensely stimulating
and warming.

- **Safety Data:** This oil may cause possible dermal sensitization on some users. If pregnant, consult a healthcare
  practitioner before use.

**Benzoin** (*Styrax Benzoin*) has a sweet, warm, vanilla-like aroma.
The sweet resin is widely used as a fixative in perfumes but has
also been used medicinally for respiratory ailments and skin
conditions such as acne, eczema, and psoriasis.

- **Chemical Families:** Esters 80%, Aldehydes 2%, Oxides
  17%, and Other 1%.
- **Therapeutic Properties:** Its main constituent is benzo-
  ic acid, which has properties that are antiseptic, antidepressant, anti-infectious, anti-inflammatory, carminative, deodorant, diuretic, and expectorant.
- **Safety Data:** Benzoin is non-toxic and non-irritant, but is
  a mild sensitizer and should be avoided if you have aller-
  gy-prone skin.

**Bergamot** (*Citrus bergamia*) is used in many skincare creams and
lotions because of its refreshing citrus nature. It is ideal for helping to calm inflamed skin and is an ingredient in some creams
for eczema and psoriasis. Bergamot's chemical makeup has antiseptic properties, which help ward off infection, cleanse
wounds, and aid in recovery. It is a favorite oil of aromathera-
pists in treating depression. Bergamot is also effective as an antispasmodic, helps to reduce leg cramps, and is used for restless

leg syndrome. It is also suitable for coughs and works as a digestive aid. Other applications include colic, flatulence, indigestion, cold sores, chickenpox, and shingles. It relieves anxiety due to its uplifting quality. It regulates appetite and helps with cystitis, UTI symptoms, herpes, acne, and oily skin.

- **Chemical Families:** Esters 31%, Monoterpenes 65%, Sesquiterpenes 0.86%, Aldehydes 0.53%, and Monoterpenols 3%.

- **Therapeutic Properties:** Analgesic, anti-anxiety, antidepressant, antiseptic, antibiotic, anti-infectious, anti-inflammatory, antispasmodic, antiviral, calmative, carminative, cicatrisant, CNS tonic, deodorant, digestive stimulant, energizing, febrifuge, sedative, stomachic, tonic, vermifuge, and vulnerary.

- **Safety Data:** Bergamot essential oil has phototoxic properties; therefore, exposure to the sun must be avoided after use. It may also interfere with the activity of certain prescription drugs.

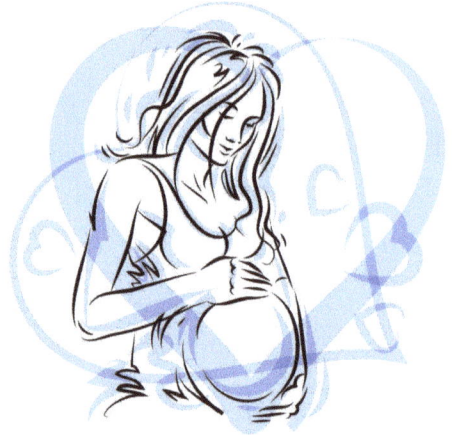

**Black Pepper** *(Piper nigrum)* is used in the treatment of pain, rheumatism, chills, flu, colds, nausea, poor circulation, exhaustion, muscular aches, and for stimulating the appetite. Black pepper is an extremely powerful anti-inflammatory agent. It enhances alertness and stamina, helps with poor circulation, aids with brain health, decreases muscular discomfort, muscle cramps, and aching muscles, and gets sluggish digestion moving again such as constipation.

- **Chemical Families:** Sesquiterpenes 37%, Monoterpenes 57%, Alcohols 2%, Oxides 0.66%, and Other 3%.

- **Therapeutic Properties:** Analgesic, antiseptic, antispasmodic, antitoxic, aphrodisiac, antiemetic, antiviral, digestive, diuretic, expectorant, febrifuge, rubefacient, warming, cognitive support, and stimulating.

- **Safety Data:** Avoid oxidized oil. This oil may cause irritation to sensitive skin and if used too much could overstimulate the kidneys.

**Virginian Cedarwood** *(Juniperus virginiana)* has been used to calm nervous tension and states of anxiety. It is useful as an expectorant, mildly astringent and treats hemorrhoids. Virginian cedarwood works well in deterring moths and other insects. It is known to help with dandruff, hair loss, and oily hair. It has been used in products formulated to relieve muscle and joint pain, preparations for acne, and hair products.

- **Chemical Families:** Sesquiterpenes 75%, Sesquiterpenols 19%, Oxides 0.57%, Ketones 0.47%, and Other 5%.

- **Therapeutic Properties:** It is a potent antiseptic, fungicidal, anti-infectious, astringent, anti-seborrhoeic, CNS tonic, diuretic, expectorant, insect repellant, mucolytic, and vein tonic.

- **Safety Data:** This oil is considered non-toxic and non-irritant. Do not use if you have a history of kidney disease.

**German Chamomile** (*Matricaria recutita*) is a relaxing and rejuvenating agent that calms nerves, reduces stress, and aids with insomnia. It can assist with cuts, wounds, and insect bites and works as an excellent skin cleanser. Chamomile is nourishing for dry and itchy skin, eases puffiness and strengthens tissues. German chamomile is known to smooth out broken capillaries, thus improving skin elasticity.

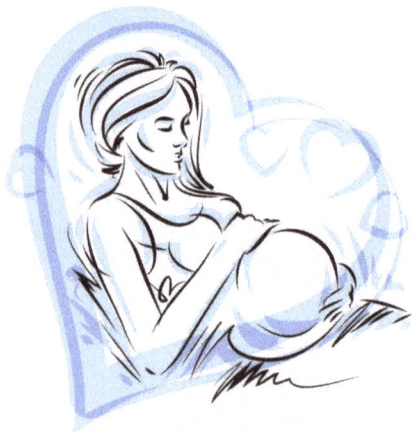

- **Chemical Families:** Sesquiterpenes 59%, Oxides 24%, Ethers 8.55%, Sesquiterpenols 3%, Ketones 1%, Monoterpenes 1%, and Other 2.54%.

- **Therapeutic Properties:** Analgesic, anti-allergic, anti-convulsant, antidepressant, antiseptic, antispasmodic, anti-inflammatory, cholagogue, diuretic, emmenagogue, febrifuge, hepatic, nervine, sedative, splenetic, stomachic, sudorific, tonic, vermifuge, and vasoconstrictor.

- **Safety Data:** While German chamomile is considered non-toxic and non-irritant, it could cause dermatitis in some individuals. This oil is not recommended for people who suffer from allergies to ragweed.

**Roman Chamomile** (*Chamaemelum nobilis*) is effective for skin care for most skin types, acne, boils, burns, eczema, inflamed or sensitive skin conditions, wounds, menstrual pain, premenstrual syndrome, headache, insomnia, restless leg syndrome, anxiety, allergies, asthma, and nervous tension. Chamomile is gentle enough for teething and colic for baby and indigestion and diarrhea for mom. It is used commercially in shampoos for fair hair as it can lighten hair color. On an emotional level, this oil is calming and soothes the spirit.

- **Chemical Families:** Esters 70%, Sesquiterpenes 4%, Monoterpenes 10%, and Alcohols 16%.

- **Therapeutic Properties:** Analgesic, antispasmodic, anti-septic, antibiotic, anti-inflammatory, anti-infectious, antidepressant, antineuralgic, antiphlogistic, bactericidal, carminative, cholagogue, cicatrizant, digestive, emmenagogue, febrifuge, hepatic, nervine, sedative, stomachic, sudorific, tonic, vermifuge, and vulnerary.

- **Safety Data:** Non-toxic, non-irritating, and non-sensitizing. This oil should not be used by anyone who is allergic to ragweed.

**Copaiba** (*Copaifera reticulata or officinalis*) has been used to treat skin hemorrhoids, diarrhea, urinary tract infections, constipation, and bronchitis. Copaiba balsam may have a "water pill" effect as it is diuretic. Chemicals in copaiba balsam make it effective at killing germs, decreasing swelling and inflammation, and loosening chest congestion due to its expectorant properties. In combination with other essential oils, it is an excellent fixative to bind more volatile aromas and extend their shelf life.

- **Chemical Families:** Sesquiterpenes 96%, Sesquiterpenols 1.5%, Oxides 1.42%, and Other 1%.

- **Therapeutic Properties:** Analgesic, antibacterial, antifungal, anti-inflammatory, antiseptic, cicatrisant, cooling, decongestant, diuretic, expectorant, immunostimulant, and calming for the nervous system.

- **Safety Data:** This oil may cause possible dermal sensitization on some users.

**Clary Sage** (*Salvia sclarea*) can be used as a deodorant, antidepressant, and a sedative. It is effective in combating oily hair and is a superior oil for acne, wrinkles, and fine lines. Women experiencing hormonal changes or menopause symptoms such as hot flashes find this oil quite beneficial. This oil should be avoided during pregnancy because of its therapeutic actions mimicking a woman's hormones but can be safely used during delivery and postpartum.

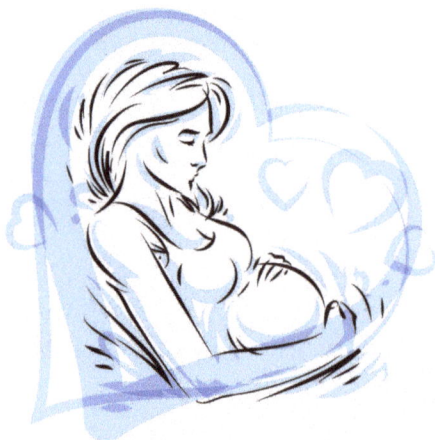

- **Chemical Families:** Esters 72%, Sesquiterpenes 3%, Alcohols 14%, and Other 11%.

- **Therapeutic Properties:** Antidepressant, anticonvulsant, antispasmodic, antiseptic, aphrodisiac, astringent, bactericidal, carminative, deodorant, digestive, emmenagogue, euphoric, hypotensive, nervine, sedative, stomachic, uterine and nerve tonic.

- **Safety Data:** Clary sage oil is non-toxic and non-sensitizing. Do not use during pregnancy. If you are at risk for breast cancer, do not use—it is unknown of the estrogen-like effect on the body.

**Coriander** (*Coriandrum sativum*) relieves mental fatigue, migraine pain, stress, and nervous debility. Coriander's warming effect helps alleviate pain, such as rheumatism, arthritis, colic, fatigue, gout, indigestion, nausea, and muscle spasms.

- **Chemical Families:** Esters 2%, Ketones 4%, Monoterpenes 9%, Alcohols 81%, and Other 4%.
- **Therapeutic Properties:** Analgesic, aperitif, aphrodisiac, antispasmodic, bactericidal, carminative, depurative, deodorant, digestive, fungicidal, revitalizing, stimulating, and stomachic.
- **Safety Data:** This oil is non-toxic, non-irritating, and non-sensitizing.

**Cypress** (*Cupressus sempervirens*) is used to prevent excessive perspiration, particularly in the feet. It is good for hemorrhoids, oily skin, and acts as an astringent in skincare applications. It is incredibly gentle and suitable for all skin types. It is ideal for various female problems and good for coughs and bronchitis. Cypress assists with varicose veins and bodily fluids by improving circulation. Other uses include edema, hemorrhoids, hot flashes, and PMS symptoms. On an emotional level, cypress offers strength, harmony, and serenity. This oil calms and soothes anger while having a positive effect on one's mood.

- **Chemical Families:** Monoterpenes 87%, Esters 2.39%, Sesquiterpenes 1.68%, Monoterpenols 1.5%, Sesquiterpenols 0.40%, Oxides 0.05%, Ketones 0.02%, Phenols 0.01%, and

Other 6.5%.

- **Therapeutic Properties:** Antibacterial, anti-infectious, anti-inflammatory, antirheumatic, antiseptic, antispasmodic, astringent, decongestant, deodorant, diuretic, hemostatic, hepatic, styptic, sudorific, venous decongestant, and vein tonic.

- **Safety Data:** Non-toxic, non-irritating, and non-sensitizing. Avoid long-term use with high blood pressure.

**Dill Weed** (*Anethum graveolens L.*) is a stimulating, revitalizing, restoring, purifying, and balancing oil. Dill is good for the digestive system and helps relieve cramps, diarrhea, flatulence, indigestion, and is known to whet the appetite.

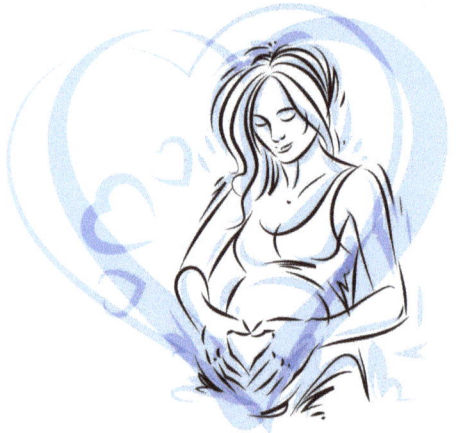

- **Chemical Families:** Ketones 54%, Monoterpenes 41%, Monoterpenols 0.36%, Ethers 0.36%, Phenols 0.20%, and Other 4%.

- **Therapeutic Properties:** Antispasmodic, carminative, digestive, disinfectant, galactagogue, sedative, stomachic, and sudorific.

- **Safety Data:** Dill weed is non-toxic and non-irritating.

**Eucalyptus** (*Eucalyptus globulus, smithii or radiata*) is used for all types of skin ailments such as burns, blisters, wounds, insect bites, lice, and skin infections. This oil is effective in combating the effects of colds and flu and is perfect for sore muscles and joints.

- **Chemical Families:** Oxides 68%, Monoterpenes 14%, Monoterpenols 14%, Esters 1%, Aldehydes 0.19%, Sesquiterpenes 0.15%, and Other 2%.

- **Therapeutic Properties:** Anti-inflammatory, antispasmodic, decongestant, deodorant, antiseptic, antibacterial, and stimulating.

- **Safety Data:** It is non-irritant and non-sensitive. Some varieties are considered toxic if taken internally. Avoid if you have high blood pressure or epilepsy. It should be used in dilution. Please check with your healthcare provider prior to use during pregnancy. Avoid use while nursing.

**Fir Needle** (*Abies sibirica*) is a popular oil used in men's fragrances, bath preparations, air fresheners, herbal oils, soaps, and shaving creams. Siberian fir is good for the sinuses, arthritic pain, rheumatism, and other aches and pains, especially if caused by inflammation.

- **Chemical Families:** Monoterpenes 65.73%, Sesquiterpenes 1.25%, Monoterpenols 3.15%, Sesquiterpenols 0.22%, Aldehydes 0.11%, Ketones 0.54%, and Esters 26.15%.

- **Therapeutic Properties:** Anti-inflammatory, antirheumatic, antispasmodic, antiseptic, deodorant, decongestant, and rubefacient, which increases local blood circulation as this oil is warming.

- **Safety Data:** Do not use this oil undiluted topically as it may cause contact dermatitis. It is non-toxic, usually non-irritant, and non-sensitizing.

**Frankincense** (*Boswellia carterii*) is highly prized in the aromatherapy industry. It is frequently used in skincare products as it is considered a valuable ingredient having remarkable anti-aging, rejuvenating, and healing properties for dry skin and wrinkles. It is beneficial for anxiety, nervous tension, asthma, and bronchitis. On an emotional level, frankincense is good for stress, irritability, and restlessness because it calms the mind.

- **Chemical Families:** Esters 1%, Monoterpenes 90%, Monoterpenols 1.65%, Sesquiterpenols 0.63%, Ketones 0.49%, Sesquiterpenes 0.36%, and Other 6%.

- **Therapeutic Properties:** Antiseptic, astringent, carminative, cicatrisant, cytophylactic, diuretic, emmenagogue, expectorant, sedative, uterine, and vulnerary.

- **Safety Data:** This oil is non-toxic, non-irritating, and non-sensitizing.

**Geranium** (*Pelargonium graveolens*) has a tremendous all-over balancing effect on the skin, creating a balance between oily and dry skin and works wonders for wrinkles. Geranium works well as a decent overall skin cleanser and makes a fabulous oil for mature and troubled skin, bringing a radiant glow to your complexion. It is indicated for disturbed

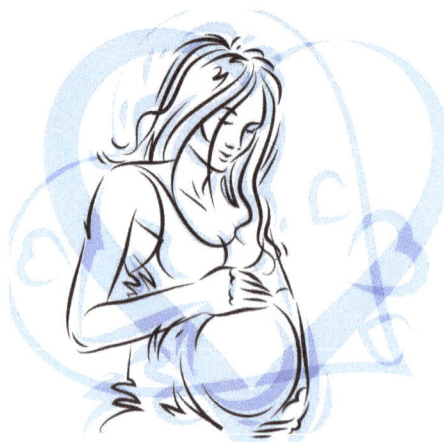

and sensitive skin, as well as broken capillaries. Geranium works well in reducing edema and fluid retention, promoting circulation, and has a stimulating effect on the lymphatic system. This oil also wards off mosquitos and head lice. Geranium is well tolerated by most individuals, but since it helps in balancing the hormonal system, care must be taken during pregnancy. On an emotional level, it calms the mind and eases frustration and irritability. Other uses include stress, nervous tension, depression, headaches, and anxiety.

- **Chemical Families:** Monoterpenes 49%, Esters 13%, Ketones 7%, Sesquiterpenes 5%, Oxides 2%, Sesquiterpenols 1%, and Other 23%.

- **Therapeutic Properties:** Antidepressant, antiseptic, astringent, antispasmodic, anti-infectious, cicatrisant, cytophylactic, diuretic, deodorant, hemostatic, styptic, tonic, vermifuge, and vulnerary.

- **Safety Data:** This oil is non-toxic, non-irritating, and non-sensitizing. Avoid use during the first and second trimester of pregnancy. Do not use if you have a history of estrogen-dependent cancer or are hypoglycemic.

**Ginger** (*Zingiber officinale*) is excellent for colds and flu, nausea (including motion sickness and morning sickness), rheumatism, coughs, and circulation issues. It has warming properties that help to relieve muscular cramps, spasms, aches, and eases stiffness in joints. It may irritate sensitive skin. Other uses include stimulating the circulatory system for poor circulation, cardiac fatigue, angina, abdominal distension, poor digestion, flatulence, rheumatism, arthritis, muscular pain, catarrh, coughs, sinusitis, and sore throats. On an emotional level, ginger increases determination and motivation.

- **Chemical Families:** Sesquiterpenes 57%, Monoterpenes 23%, Aldehydes 5%, Oxides 3%, Monoterpenols 3%, Sesquiterpenols 3%, Ketones 1%, and Other 5%.

- **Therapeutic Properties:** Analgesic, anti-inflammatory, antiemetic, antiseptic, antispasmodic, carminative, diaphoretic, expectorant, febrifuge, heart tonic, laxative, rubefacient, stimulant, stomachic, sudorific, and tonic.

- **Safety Data:** It is non-irritating and non-toxic, but may be sensitizing to some people.

**Grapefruit** (*Citrus x paradisi*) is spiritually uplifting, eases muscle fatigue and stiffness, relieves nervous exhaustion, and alleviates depression. It helps to clear congested, oily, and acne-prone skin. Grapefruit is sometimes added to creams and lotions as a natural toner and cellulite treatment.

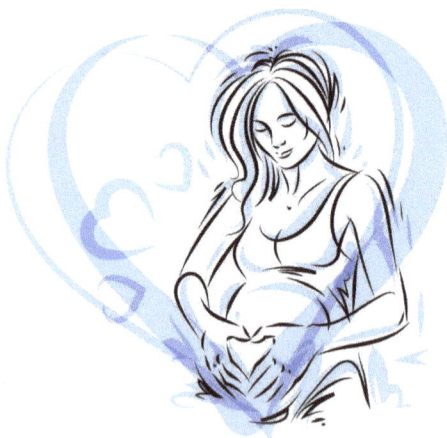

- **Chemical Families:** Monoterpenes 94%, Oxides 1.6%, Monoterpenols 1%, Aldehydes 0.60%, Ketones 0.37%, and Other 2.56%.

- **Therapeutic Properties:** Antiviral, astringent, antidepressant, antiseptic, decongestant, diuretic, and tonic.

- **Safety Data:** It is non-toxic and non-irritating for most individuals. It can cause photosensitivity.

**Helichrysum** (*Helichrysum italicum*) is an effective oil for acne, bruises, boils, burns, cuts, dermatitis, eczema, irritated skin, and wounds. It supports the body through post-viral fatigue and convalescence, and can also be used to repair skin damaged by psoriasis, eczema, or ulceration.

- **Chemical Families:** Oxides 33.51%, Monoterpenes 26.31%, Sesquiterpenes 24%, Sesquiterpenols 4%, Monoterpenols 3%, and Other 9%.

- **Therapeutic Properties:** Anti-inflammatory, antibacterial, analgesic, antiseptic, antispasmodic, antifungal, antiviral, antimicrobial, and a tonic for the nervous system.

- **Safety Data:** This oil is non-toxic, non-irritating, and non-sensitizing. Please check with your healthcare provider before using during pregnancy.

**Jasmine** (*Jasminum grandiflorum*) is a sensual, soothing, calming oil that promotes love and peace. It is necessary to note that all absolutes are highly concentrated by nature. The complexity of the fragrance, particularly the rare and exotic notes, is well-regarded for its aphrodisiac properties. Other uses include nervous anxiety, restlessness, depression, stimulation, to strengthen contractions, ease labor pain, and help propel afterbirth. On an emotional level, this oil is a favorite for lifting one's spirit from depression, apathy, and weakness.

- **Chemical Families:** Esters 52%, Diterpenols 13%, Monoterpenols 10%, Triterpenes 10%, Phenols 2%, Ketones

1.72%, Monoterpenes 1%, Sesquiterpenols 0.56%, and Other 3%.

- **Therapeutic Properties:** Antidepressant, antiseptic, antispasmodic, aphrodisiac, expectorant, galactagogue, parturient, sedative, and uterine.

- **Safety Data:** It is non-irritating, non-sensitizing, and non-toxic; but may be allergenic. Avoid use during the first and second trimester of pregnancy.

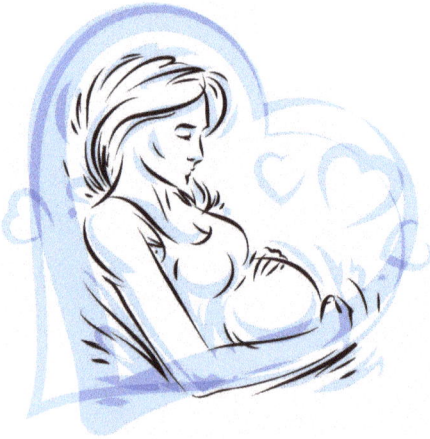

**Juniper Berry** (*Juniperus communis*) is a supportive, restoring, and tonic aid. It is used in acne treatments, for oily skin, dermatitis, weeping eczema, psoriasis, and blocked pores. It is considered purifying and clearing. It returns skin tissue to normal functioning.

- **Chemical Families:** Monoterpenes 76%, Sesquiterpenes 23%, Sesquiterpenols 0.65%, Monoterpenols 0.42%, and Oxides 0.38%.

- **Therapeutic Properties:** Antiseptic, antirheumatic, antispasmodic, astringent, carminative, depurative, diuretic, rubefacient, stimulating, stomachic, sudorific, vulnerary, and tonic.

- **Safety Data:** Juniper berry is non-irritating and non-sensitizing. Avoid if you have a history of kidney disease or high blood pressure.

**Lavandin** (*Lavandula intermedia*) is considered one of the most useful and versatile essential oils for easing sore muscles and joints, relieving muscle stiffness, clearing the lungs and sinuses from phlegm, and healing wounds and dermatitis. Lavandin is advantageous for burns and healing of the skin. Its antiseptic and analgesic properties aid with easing pain and preventing infection. Lavandin's cytophylactic properties promote rapid healing and help reduce scarring. Its calming scent reduces anxiety and promotes sleep.

- **Chemical Families:** Esters 34.46%, Ketones 6.41%, Monoterpenes 6.71%, Monoterpenols 5.62%, Oxides 3.79%, Sesquiterpenes 3.24%, and Sesquiterpenols 0.85%.

- **Therapeutic Properties:** Analgesic, anticonvulsant, antidepressant, antiphlogistic, antirheumatic, antiseptic, antispasmodic, antiviral, bactericidal, carminative, cholagogue, cicatrisant, cordial, cytophylactic, decongestant, deodorant, diuretic, expectorant, nervine, and vulnerary.

- **Safety Data:** It is non-toxic, non-irritating, and non-sensitizing. Do not use during the first trimester of pregnancy.

**Lavender** (*Lavandula angustifolia*) is most commonly used for burns and the healing of the skin. It has antiseptic and analgesic properties that ease the pain of a burn and prevents infection. Lavender also has cytophylactic properties that promote rapid healing and reduce scarring. Lavender does an excellent job at balancing oil production in the skin as well as clearing blemishes, evening skin tone, and even helping to hydrate dry skin. Lavender is indicated for all skin types and can be used at any step in your skincare regimen. Lavender is beneficial for colds, flu, bronchitis, throat infections, asthma, high blood pressure, and migraines. It is also excellent for helping with insomnia. Other uses include pain, inflammation, dermatitis, eczema, psoriasis, boils, wounds, sunburn, sunstroke, muscular aches/pains, sciatica, rheumatism, arthritis, stress, mental/emotional agitation, depression, anxiety, headaches, PMS, menstrual pain, catarrh, and bug bites. On an emotional level, it helps calm the mind, comfort feelings, alleviate fears, and revive the spirit, as it is very soothing to the inner man.

- **Chemical Families:** Esters 41%, Monoterpenols 35%, Monoterpenes 10%, Oxides 1%, Ketones 0.15%, and Other 12%.

- **Therapeutic Properties:** Analgesic, anticonvulsant, antidepressant, antiphlogistic, antirheumatic, antiseptic, antispasmodic, antiviral, bactericide, carminative, cholagogue, cicatrisant, cordial, cytophylactic, decongestant, deodorant, diuretic, emmenagogue, fungicide, hypotensive, nervine, restorative, sedative, sudorific, and vulnerary.

- **Safety Data:** Non-toxic, non-irritating, and non-sensitizing. Do not use during the first trimester of pregnancy.

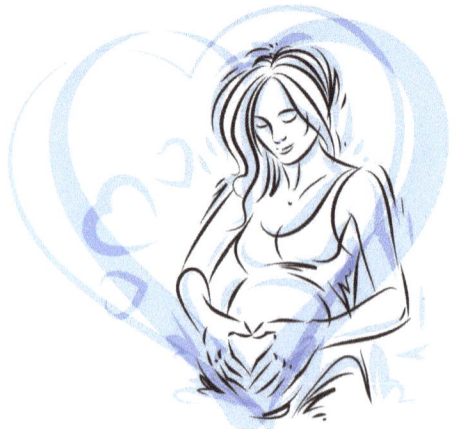

**Lemon** (*Citrus x limon*) is recognized as a cleanser and antiseptic with refreshing and cooling properties. For the skin and hair, lemon is used for its cleansing effect, as well as for treating cuts, boils, and acne. This oil's fresh scent is treasured for improving concentration, reducing acidity in the body while assisting with digestion and eliminating cellulite, rheumatism, arthritis, and gout. It is beneficial for the circulatory system and aids with blood flow, reduces blood pressure, and helps with nosebleeds. Lemon oil can be used to help reduce a fever, relieve throat infections, bronchitis, and heal cold sores, herpes, and insect bites. Other uses include stimulating the immune system. On an emotional level, lemon alleviates fear and uplifts the spirit.

- **Chemical Families:** Monoterpenes 96%, Sesquiterpenes 0.10%, Monoterpenols 0.14%, Aldehydes 1.92%, Ketones 0.07%, Esters 0.82%, and Oxides 0.20%.

- **Therapeutic Properties:** Antimicrobial, anti-anemic, antirheumatic, antiseptic, antispasmodic, astringent, anti-sclerotic, bactericidal, carminative, cicatrisant, depurative, detoxification, diaphoretic, diuretic, febrifuge, hemostatic, hypotensive, insecticidal, rubefacient, tonic, and vermifuge.

- **Safety Data:** Non-toxic and non-irritating, although it is phototoxic and should be avoided before exposure to direct sunlight. Lemon may cause skin irritation for some.

**Lemongrass** (*Cymbopogon flexuosus*) is known for its invigorating qualities and makes an excellent antidepressant. It can be used in facial toners as its astringent properties help fight acne and oily skin. Lemongrass tones and fortifies the nervous system and can be used in the bath for soothing muscular nerves and pain. Lemongrass has an outstanding reputation for keeping insects away, controlling perspiration and for treating athlete's foot. This oil relieves the symptoms of jet lag, helps with nervousness and anxiety, and clears headaches. It is useful with respiratory conditions such as sore throats, laryngitis, and fever and helps prevent the spreading of infectious diseases when diffused. It is also good for colitis, indigestion, and gastroenteritis.

- **Chemical Families:** Aldehydes 83.50%, Monoterpenols 4.02%, Monoterpenes 3.57%, Ketones 2.15%, Sesquiterpenes 2.10%, Oxides 1.15%, Esters 0.43%, Phenols 0.24%, and Other 2.84%.

- **Therapeutic Properties:** Analgesic, antidepressant, antimicrobial, antipyretic, antiseptic, astringent, bactericidal, carminative, deodorant, diuretic, febrifuge, fungicidal, galactagogue, insecticidal, nervine, nervous system sedative, and tonic.

- **Safety Data:** Avoid use with individuals with glaucoma and with children. Use caution in prostatic hyperplasia and with skin hypersensitivity or damaged skin. Avoid use during the first trimester of pregnancy. Avoid if you have a history of high blood pressure.

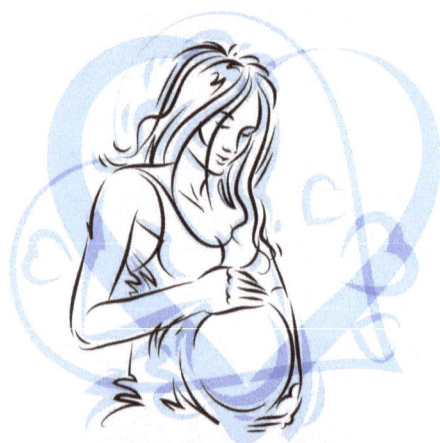

**Lime** (*Citrus aurantifolia*) has a crisp, refreshing citrus scent with uplifting and revitalizing properties that help with depression. It acts as an astringent on the skin and helps clear oily skin. Lime cools fevers due to colds and flu, eases coughs and strengthens the immune system as well as treats bronchitis, asthma, and sinusitis. Lime oil is also helpful for arthritis, rheumatism, poor circulation, and in eliminating cellulite and obesity.

- **Chemical Families:** Aldehydes 0.4%, Esters 0.2%, Ketones 0.8%, Monoterpenes 76.5%, Monoterpenol 11.42%, Oxides 1.77%, Sesquiterpenes 3.93%, and Sesquiterpenols 0.01%.

- **Therapeutic Properties:** Antiseptic, antiviral, astringent, aperitif, bactericidal, disinfectant, febrifuge, hemostatic, restorative, and tonic.

- **Safety Data:** Lime is considered phototoxic; users should avoid direct sunlight after application.

**Mandarin** (*Citrus reticulata*) is often used as a digestive aid and to ease anxiety. It is commonly used in soaps, cosmetics, perfumes, and colognes. This tangy oil is used to increase circulation to the skin, prevent stretch marks, and reduce fluid retention. Mandarin has many applications in the flavoring industry. It is good for upset stomach for children and flatulence. On an emotional level, mandarin is considered a happy oil. It brightens the spirit, relieving stress, and anxiety.

- **Chemical Families:** Monoterpenes 97.9%, Sesquiterpenes 0.22%, and Monoterpenols 0.63%.

- **Therapeutic Properties:** Antiseptic, antispasmodic, carminative, cholagogue, cytophylactic, depurative, digestive, diuretic, sedative, stomachic, and tonic.

- **Safety Data:** Non-toxic, non-irritating, and non-sensitizing. Direct sunlight should be avoided after use as it may be phototoxic.

**Marjoram** (*Origanum majorana*) is a comforting oil that can be massaged into the abdomen during menstruation, or added to a warm compress to ease discomfort. It is useful for treating tired aching muscles or in a sports massage. Marjoram's pain-relieving properties are helpful for rheumatic pains, sprains, spasms, as well as for swollen joints and achy muscles. It can be added to a warm or hot bath at the first sign of a cold. This oil is helpful for asthma and other respiratory complaints and has a calming effect on emotions, especially for hyperactive people. It soothes the digestive system and helps with indigestion, constipation, and flatulence. Marjoram is superb as a relaxant and is useful for headaches, migraines, and insomnia.

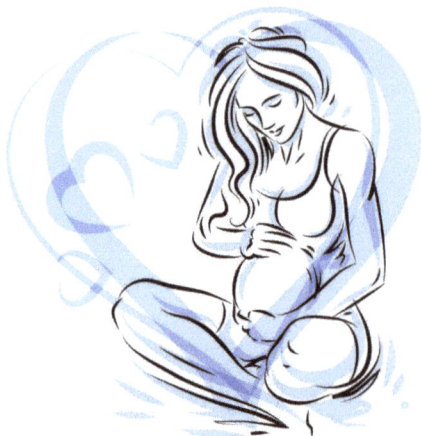

- **Chemical Families:** Monoterpenes 41.50%, Sesquiterpenes 2.65%, Monoterpenols 52.13%, Esters 2.53%, and Oxides 0.15%.

- **Therapeutic Properties:** Analgesic, antispasmodic, anaphrodisiac, antiseptic, antiviral, bactericidal, carminative, cephalic, cordial, diaphoretic, digestive, diuretic, emmenagogue, expectorant, fungicidal, hypotensive, laxative, nervine, sedative, stomachic, vasodilator, and vulnerary.

- **Safety Data:** Marjoram is generally non-toxic, non-irritating, and non-sensitizing. Use with caution if you have low blood pressure.

**Neroli** (*Citrus aurantium*) increases circulation and stimulates new cell growth. It prevents scarring and stretch marks and is useful in treating skin conditions linked to emotional stress. Any skin type can benefit from this oil, although it is particularly nourishing for dry, irritated, or sensitive skin. Neroli regulates oiliness, minimizes enlarged pores, and helps clear acne and blemished skin, especially if the skin lacks moisture. With regular treatment, it can reduce the appearance of fragile or broken capillaries and varicose veins. Neroli is useful for dry, sensitive, and mature skin as it helps improves elasticity. It is also known to help relieve muscle spasms and heart palpitations, hypertension, digestive spasms, diarrhea, nervous tension, insomnia, anxiety, and depression. On an emotional level, this oil helps bring clarity and focus.

- **Chemical Families:** Monoterpenols 43.96%, Monoterpenes 36.51%, Esters 9.59%, Sesquiterpenols 9.11%, and Other 0.65%.

- **Therapeutic Properties:** Antidepressant, antiseptic, anti-infectious, antispasmodic, aphrodisiac, bactericidal, carminative, cicatrisant, cytophylactic, cordial, deodorant, digestive, nervine, sedative, and tonic.

- **Safety Data:** Non-toxic, non-irritating, and non-sensitizing.

**Sweet Orange** (*Citrus sinensis*) helps with dull skin, the flu, gums, and stress. This oil is truly uplifting, excellent for stress while calming digestive problems and eliminating toxins. It stimulates the lymphatic system and supports the formation of collagen in the skin.

- **Chemical Families:** Aldehydes 8.71%, Monoterpenes 98.67%, Monoterpenols 0.168%, and Sesquiterpenes 0.025%.

- **Therapeutic Properties:** anti-anxiety, antibacterial, antidepressant, antiseptic, antispasmodic, antiviral, aphrodisiac, carminative, deodorant, digestive stimulant and tonic, disinfectant, energizing, liver supporter, stomachic, nervous system stimulant, and tonic for the cardiac and circulatory systems.

- **Safety Data:** It is considered phototoxic; therefore, exposure to sunlight after use should be avoided.

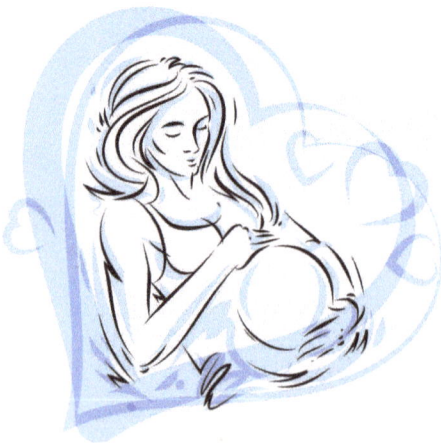

**Palmarosa** (*Cymbopogon martini*) is used extensively as a fragrance component in cosmetics, perfumes and especially soaps due to its excellent tenacity. It also works fantastic as a disinfectant. Palmarosa is effective in treating acne surface scars and wrinkles caused by prolonged exposure to the sun. It delivers exceptional hydration to the skin, and some research demonstrates its ability to renew skin cells and assist in the regulation of sebum production. This oil can be diffused to prevent the spread of flu, viral infections, and bacteria. It is also beneficial for heart palpitations, aches, and pains, insomnia, and anxiety.

- **Chemical Families:** Monoterpenes 2.24%, Sesquiterpenes 2.33%, Monoterpenols 72.85%, Sesquiterpenols 1.09%, Aldehydes 4.72%, Esters 10.26%, Oxides 0.31%, and Phenols 0.06%.

- **Therapeutic Properties:** Antifungal, anti-infectious, anti-inflammatory, analgesic, antiseptic, antispasmodic, bactericidal, cicatrisant, digestive, febrifuge, hydrating, digestive stimulant, circulatory stimulant, and tonic.

- **Safety Data:** Palmarosa is a dermal irritant. Please consult your healthcare provider before use during pregnancy. Avoid if you have a history of high blood pressure.

**Patchouli** (*Pogostemon cablin*) is beneficial for combating nervous disorders, nausea, helping with dandruff, sores, skin irritations, and acne. Patchouli has been shown to stimulate cell regeneration. It is superb for mature, dry, and chapped skin. In the perfumery industry, patchouli improves with age, and the aged product is what is preferred over freshly harvested. In aromatherapy, it is an excellent fixative that can help extend other, more expensive oils.

- **Chemical Families:** Sesquiterpenes 58.15%, Sesquiterpenols 37.38%, Oxides 1.87%, Ketones 0.76%, Monoterpenes 0.39%, and Other 1.45%.

- **Therapeutic Properties:** Antidepressant, anti-inflammatory, antimicrobial, antiseptic, antitoxic, antiviral, aphrodisiac, astringent, bactericidal, deodorant, diuretic, fungicidal, nervine, prophylactic, stimulating, and tonic.

- **Safety Data:** No known cautions.

**Peppermint** (*Mentha x piperita*) has long been credited as being useful in combating stomach ailments and soothing the digestive system. It's excellent for headaches, travel sickness, and jet lag. It is viewed as an antispasmodic and antimicrobial agent. Most people know it as a flavoring or scenting agent in food, beverages, skin, and hair care products (where it has a cooling effect by constricting capillaries). It helps with bruises and sore joints.

- **Chemical Families:** Monoterpenes 5.43%, Sesquiterpenes 2.26%, Monoterpenols 37.58%, Ketones 32.88%, Esters 4.38%, Oxides 6.19%, and Ethers 4.37%.

- **Therapeutic Properties:** Antifungal, antiseptic, antispasmodic, astringent, anti-inflammatory, analgesic, carminative, febrifuge, decongestant, expectorant, and stimulating to the circulatory and immune systems.

- **Safety Data:** Peppermint can be sensitizing due to the menthol content. Do not use if you have cardiac fibrillation. Avoid if you have a history of high blood pressure. This oil is considered safe during pregnancy but should be avoided while nurs-

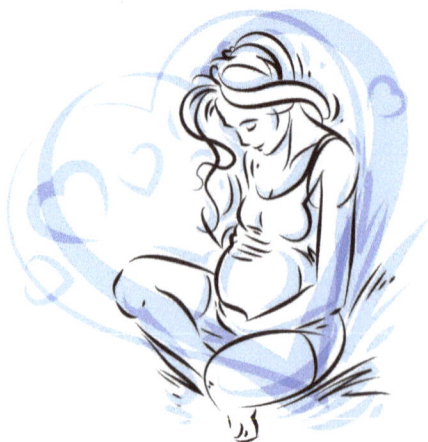

ing. May reduce milk supply when breastfeeding.

**Petitgrain** (*Citrus aurantium sp. amara*) is believed to have up-lifting properties and is used for calming anger and stress. It is commonly used in the skincare industry for acne, oily skin, and as a deodorizing agent. Petitgrain is valued for its ability to reduce pain and spasms in the lower intestines. Its calming qualities make it a favorite for insomnia.

- **Chemical Families:** Esters 54.49%, Monoterpenols 35.04%, Monoterpenes 9.14%, and Other 1.33%.

- **Therapeutic Properties:** Analgesic, anti-anxiety, antibacterial, anticonvulsant, antidepressant, antifungal, antimicrobial, anti-inflammatory, antioxidant, antiseptic, antispasmodic, antiviral, calming, cooling, deodorant, hypotensive, immuno-support, and nervine. It's a stimulant, tonic, and sedative for the nervous system.

- **Safety Data:** Petitgrain is generally considered non-toxic, non-irritant, and non-sensitizing.

**Pine** (*Pinus sylvestris*) is good as a circulatory agent, decongestant and deodorant. Pine is valued as extraordinary for the respiratory system, helping with decongestion. It has been applied to eczema, cuts, lice, muscular aches, neuralgia, psoriasis, rheumatism, ringworm, scrapes, and sinusitis.

- **Chemical Families:** Monoterpenes 90.83%, Sesquiterpenes 4.30%, Monoterpenols 1.48%, Esters 0.67%, and Oxides 0.98%.

- **Therapeutic Properties:** Anti-inflammatory, analgesic, antibacterial, antibiotic, antifungal, antiseptic, antiviral, antirheumatic, antispasmodic, decongestant, expectorant, pain reliever, rubefacient, and warming.

- **Safety Data:** Pine is considered safe since it is non-toxic and non-irritant but should be used with caution on the skin since it can cause irritation in high doses and may sensitize the skin.

**Rosalina** (*Melaleuca ericifolia*) is well known for its antiseptic, spasmolytic and anticonvulsant properties. It works great for upper respiratory tract congestion and infections and acts as a gentle expectorant, especially with small children. Rosalina has anti-infectious properties and helps to deeply relax and calm individuals, which may be under pressure. It is useful for insomnia and other sleep disorders. This oil has been traditionally used for acne, boils, and herpes. It is very mild and safe on most skin types and great for children.

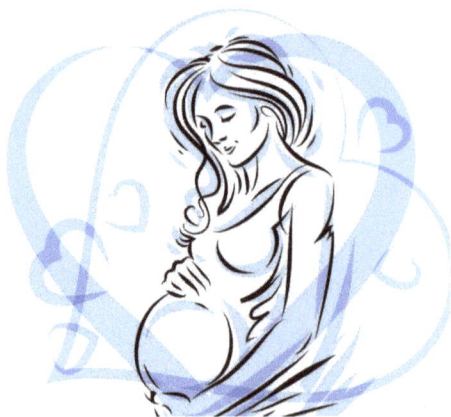

- **Chemical Families:** Monoterpenes 22.8%, Sesquiterpenes 6.62%, Monoterpenols 52.6%, Sesquiterpenols 1.5%, Esters 0.26%, and Oxides 10.24%.

- **Therapeutic Properties:** Antibacterial, antimicrobial, analgesic, anti-anxiety, cicatrisant, immunostimulant, antiviral, anti-inflammatory, and mucolytic.

- **Safety Data:** There are no known safety concerns associated with this essential oil. It is a very gentle and safe oil.

**Rose** (*Rosa damascene*) is an uplifting aphrodisiac and is wonderful for meditation. This oil is prevalent in perfumery, works as a great emollient, and is perfect for skin preparation. This oil is particularly beneficial for mature, dry, or sensitive skin with redness and inflammation. As a tonic, it has a soothing quality for inflammation and constricting action on capillaries. Rose oil lifts a sad heart and is used in the treatment of depression, grief, anger, fear, and other unpleasant emotions. It supports the heart and digestive systems and is considered one of the most incredible remedies for female problems such as balancing hormones during menopause and PMS. Rose is beneficial for palpitations, irritability, and insomnia.

- **Chemical Families:** Monoterpenols 51.27%, Sesquiterpenes 2.41%, Aldehydes 2.06%, Phenols 1.80%, Esters 1.58%, Ethers 1.45%, Monoterpenes 1.11%, Oxides 0.47%, and Other 14.90%.

- **Therapeutic Properties:** Antidepressant, antiphlogistic, antiseptic, antispasmodic, antiviral, aphrodisiac, astringent, bactericidal, choleretic, cicatrizant, depurative, emmenagogue, hemostatic, hepatic, laxative, sedative, stomachic, and tonic for the heart, liver, stomach, and uterus.

- **Safety Data:** Non-toxic, non-irritating, and non-sensitizing. Avoid use during the first trimester of pregnancy.

**Rosemary** (*Rosmarinus officinalis*) stimulates cell renewal and improves dry or mature skin, eases lines and wrinkles, and heals burns and wounds. It can clear acne, blemishes, or dull, dry skin by fighting bacteria and regulating oil secretions. This warming oil improves circulation and can reduce the appearance of broken capillaries and varicose veins. It tones and tightens the skin and is useful for sagging skin. Rosemary helps with overcoming mental fatigue and sluggishness by stimulating and strengthening the entire nervous system. It also enhances mental clarity while aiding alertness and concentration. It is beneficial to use in stressful conditions.

- **Chemical Families:** Monoterpenes 27.55%, Sesquiterpenes 3.58%, Monoterpenols 6.5%, Sesquiterpenols 0.15%, Ketones 10.97%, Esters 1.05%, and Oxides 50.15%.

- **Therapeutic Properties:** Analgesic, anti-inflammatory, antirheumatic, antiseptic, astringent, antispasmodic, antiviral, decongestant, diuretic, expectorant, restorative, and stimulant.

- **Safety Data:** Rosemary is generally non-toxic and non-sensitizing but is not suitable for people with epilepsy.

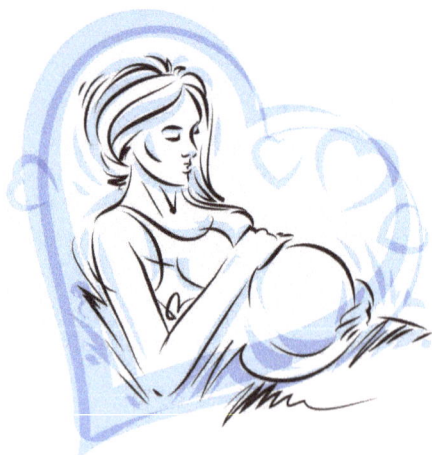

**Sandalwood** (*Santalum album*) is known to create an exotic, sensual mood with a reputation as an aphrodisiac. It is used extensively in the perfume industry as a fixative and in body care products for the fragrance it provides. In aromatherapy, sandalwood is used to help combat bronchitis, chapped and dry skin, mood disturbances, stress, and stretch marks. It is said to have anti-microbial properties, which makes it effective in treating skin conditions such as acne, oily skin, and is especially beneficial for dehydrated skin and eczema. It is also used to treat varicose veins, swollen lymph nodes, headaches, and insomnia. Sandal-wood has powerful antibacterial and antifungal agents, which makes it beneficial for respiratory infections and urinary tract infections. On an emotional level, it is good for nervous depression, fear, stress, and a hectic lifestyle.

- **Chemical Families:** Aldehydes 2.85%, Monoterpenes 0.01%, Sesquiterpenes 3.83%, and Sesquiterpenols 80.43%.

- **Therapeutic Properties:** Anti-inflammatory, antiphlogistic, antiseptic, antispasmodic, astringent, carminative, demulcent, diuretic, emollient, expectorant, sedative, and tonic

- **Safety Data:** Sandalwood is considered non-toxic, non-irritant, and non-sensitizing.

**Spearmint** (*Mentha spicata*) is used as a local or topical anesthetic. Spearmint is an uplifting oil, making it ideal for alleviating fatigue and depression. It is also reputed to relieve itching (pruritus, eczema, urticaria), cool the skin, and aid in healing wounds, sores, and scabs. This oil is terrific for the digestive system, flatulence, constipation, vomiting, nausea, and respiratory infections due to coughs, bronchitis, asthma, catarrh, and sinusitis.

- **Chemical Families:** Ketones 66.35%, Monoterpenes 19.68%, Monoterpenols 3.10%, Sesquiterpenes 2.39%, Sesquiterpenols 1.45%, Oxides 0.67%, Phenols 0.42%, and Other 4.87%.

- **Therapeutic Properties:** Antispasmodic, astringent, carminative, decongestant, digestive, diuretic, expectorant, stimulant, and restorative.

- **Safety Data:** Spearmint may irritate mucous membranes. Please check with your healthcare provider before use during the first trimester of pregnancy.

**Spruce** (*Picea mariana*) is used for the treatment of asthma, bronchitis, coughs, colds, flu, infection, muscle aches and pains, poor circulation, and respiratory weakness. Spruce is used in baths for tired muscles, room sprays, detergents, and in cough and cold preparations. It is a popular choice for arthritis and rheumatism with its powerful anti-inflammatory properties.

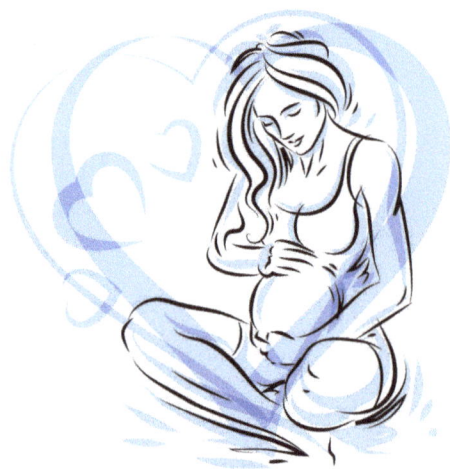

- **Chemical Families:** Monoterpenes 62.11%, Esters 34.05%, Sesquiterpenols 0.98%, Monoterpenols 2.29%, and Sesquiterpenes 6.04%.

- **Therapeutic Properties:** Anti-inflammatory, antirheumatic, antispasmodic, antiseptic, decongestant, diuretic, rubefacient, and warming.

- **Safety Data:** At low doses, it is non-toxic, non-irritating, and non–sensitizing.

**Tangerine** (*Citrus reticulata*) is a refreshing and rejuvenating oil.

Its aroma clears the mind and can help to eliminate emotional confusion. Tangerine is truly comforting, soothing, and warming oil used in perfumes and soaps. This oil is good for weeping wounds and cuts that won't heal. Its healing properties include acting as a stimulant for the lymphatic system and a tonic agent. It improves the circulation of blood and phlegm, boosts digestion, helps to maintain the balance in the skin with cicatrizant properties and aids with rashes, dryness, and cracking of the skin. Tangerine essential oil eases constipation and treats diarrhea, relieves spasms, flatulence, hair problems, and dandruff. The skin should not be exposed to sunlight after a treatment. Similarly, the oil should be diluted well before use on the skin.

- **Chemical Families:** Monoterpenes 93.83%, Monoterpenols 1.59%, Aldehydes 0.62%, Sesquiterpenes 0.35%, Ketones 0.20%, Oxides 0.16%, Esters 0.09%, and Other 2.45%.

- **Therapeutic Properties:** Anti-anxiety, antibacterial, antidepressant, antimicrobial, antioxidant, antiseptic, antispasmodic, carminative, digestive tonic, diuretic, energizing, sedative, stimulant, and tonic.

- **Safety Data:** Tangerine may show some extent of phototoxicity in certain skin types, but in general, it is non-toxic, non-irritating, and non-sensitizing.

**Tea Tree** (*Melaleuca alternifolia*) is best known as a powerful immune stimulant. It helps fight all three categories of infectious organisms, including bacterial, viral, and fungal. When used in vapor therapy, tea tree can help with colds, measles, sinusitis, and viral infections. For skin and hair, it has been used to combat acne, oily skin, head lice, and dandruff. It clears up pimples and significantly reduces their reoccurrence due to its antimicrobial and anti-inflammatory power. This oil invigorates the heart and mind, uplifts the spirit, and builds confidence. It is immune-boosting and fights thrush, vaginitis, cystitis, pruritis, chronic infections, asthma, bronchitis, catarrh, cough, sinusitis, whooping cough, acne, athlete's foot, burns, cold sores, and heals wounds.

- **Chemical Families:** Monoterpenes 48.09%, Monoterpenols 40.30%, Sesquiterpenes 7.16%, Oxides 3.99%, Sesquiterpenols 0.75%.

- **Therapeutic Properties:** antimicrobial, antifungal, antiseptic, bactericide, balsamic, cicatrisant, expectorant, fungicide, immunostimulant, insecticide, stimulant, sudorific

- **Safety Data:** This is a non-toxic and non-irritant essential oil. It could be dermally sensitizing to some individuals; beware of oxidation. Do not take internally.

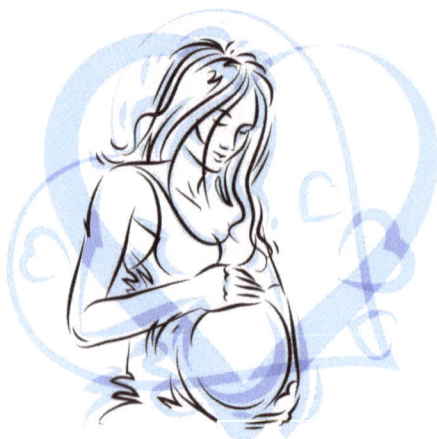

**Vetiver** (*Vetiveria zizanioides*) is believed to be deeply relaxing and comforting. It is used as a base note in perfumery and aromatherapy applications. This oil is useful in dispelling irritability, anger, and hysteria due to its relaxation qualities while having a balancing effect on the hormonal system. Vetiver helps to reduce wrinkles and stretch marks while nourishing and moisturizing the skin. It is also beneficial for helping wounds heal. The scent of this blend is believed to stimulate and strengthen the reproductive system, address the discomfort associated with menstruation, and balance hormones. It eases a stressed mind and calms emotional outbursts. It promotes concentration when you need to focus on a task. It also can boost libido when diffused due to its aphrodisiac properties, as well as address sleep disorders.

- **Chemical Families:** Sesquiterpenes 43.86%, Sesquiterpenols 14.94%, Ketones 3.01%, and Esters 0.43%.

- **Therapeutic Properties:** Antibacterial, antidepressant, aphrodisiac, antifungal, antiseptic, anti-inflammatory, circulatory stimulant, deodorant, immune support and stimulant, nervine, sedative, strengthening, tonic, cicatrizant, and vulnerary.

- **Safety Data:** No known toxicity. Avoid high concentrations during pregnancy.

**Ylang Ylang** (*Cananga odorata*) assists with problems such as high blood pressure, rapid breathing and heartbeat, nervous conditions, impotence, and frigidity. This oil is best suited for use in the perfumery and skincare industries due to it having a balancing effect on sebum and is useful for both oily and dry skin types. Other applications include palpitations, hypertension, tachycardia, anxiety, anger, shock, rage, frustration, stress, nervous tension, sexual inadequacy, PMS, mood swings, and split ends.

- **Chemical Families:** Esters 16%, Sesquiterpenes 16%, Monoterpenes 47%, and Alcohols 20%.

- **Therapeutic Properties:** Antidepressant, antisebor-rheic, antiseptic, aphrodisiac, hypotensive, nervine, and sedative.

- **Safety Data:** This oil is non-toxic, non-irritating, and non-sensitizing; overuse may cause nausea and/or head-aches. This oil is not recommended if you have low blood pressure.

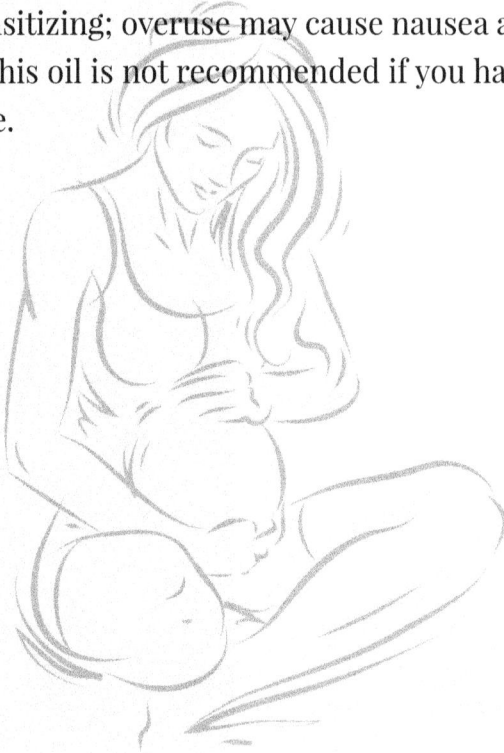

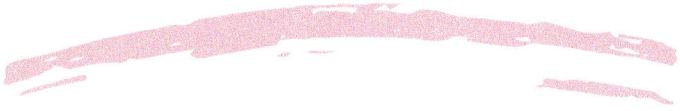

# Charts

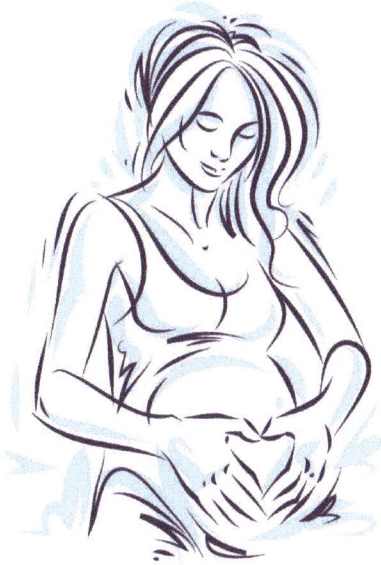

# Essential Oils Safe During Pregnancy

The oils below are used commonly during pregnancy and present no hazard. Most moms-to-be prefer citrus-smelling oils, but several other oils can be used during your pregnancy.

| | |
|---|---|
| Amyris | *Amyris balsamifera* |
| Balsam Fir | *Abies balsamea* |
| Bergamot | *Citrus bergamia* |
| Benzoin | *Styrax tonkinensis* |
| Black Pepper | *Piper nigrum* |
| Virginian Cedarwood | *Juniperus virginiana* |
| German Chamomile | *Chamomilla recutita* |
| Roman Chamomile | *Chamaemelum nobile* |
| Copaiba | *Copaifera langsdofii, Copaifera officinalis* |
| Coriander | *Coriandrum sativum* |
| Cypress | *Cupressus sempervirens* |
| Dill Weed | *Anethum graveolens* |
| Fir Needle | *Abies alba, Abies sachalinensis, Abies sibirica* |
| Frankincense | *Boswellia carterii* |
| Geranium | *Pelargonium graveolens* |
| Ginger | *Zingiber officinale* |
| Grapefruit | *Citrus paradisi* |

| | |
|---|---|
| Helichrysum | *Helichrysum italicum, Helichrysum splendidum* |
| Jasmine | *Jasminum sambac absolute, Jasminum grandiflorum* |
| Juniper Berry | *Juniperus communis* |
| Lavender | *Lavandula angustifolia* |
| Lavandin | *Lavandula x intermedia* |
| Lemon | *Citrus limon* |
| Mandarin | *Citrus reticulata* |
| Marjoram, Sweet | *Origanum majorana* |
| Neroli | *Citrus x aurantium* |
| Orange, Sweet | *Citrus sinensis* |
| Palmarosa | *Cymbopogon martini var motia* |
| Patchouli | *Pogostemon cablin* |
| Peppermint | *Mentha x piperita* |
| Petitgrain | *Citrus aurantium* |
| Pine | *Pinus Sylvestris* |
| Rosalina | *Melaleuca ericifolia* |
| Rose | *Rosa damascena* |
| Sandalwood | *Santalum album or Santalum spicatum* |
| Spearmint | *Mentha spicata* |
| Spruce | *Picea abies* |
| Tangerine | *Citrus reticulata* |
| Tea Tree | *Melaleuca alternifolia* |

| Vetiver | *Vetiveria zizanoides* |
|---------|------------------------|
| Ylang Ylang | *Cananga odorata* |

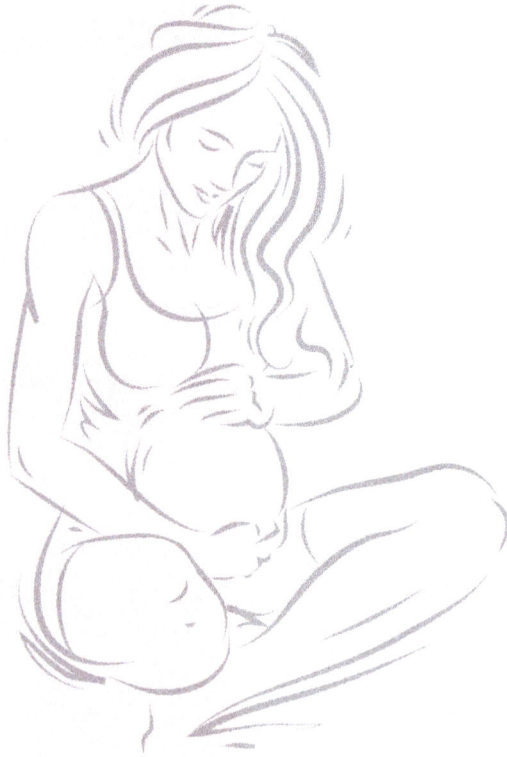

# Essential Oils for Labor

| | |
|---|---|
| Bergamot | *Citrus bergamia* |
| German Chamomile | *Chamomilla recutita* |
| Roman Chamomile | *Chamaemelum nobile* |
| Clary Sage | *Salvia sclarea* |
| Copaiba | *Copaifera langsdofii, Copaifera officinalis* |
| Cypress | *Cupressus sempervirens* |
| Eucalyptus | *Eucalyptus globulus, smithii or radiata* |
| Fir Needle | *Abies alba, Abies sachalinensis, Abies sibirica* |
| Frankincense | *Boswellia carterii* |
| Geranium | *Pelargonium graveolens* |
| Helichrysum | *Helichrysum italicum, Helichrysum splendidum* |
| Jasmine | *Jasminum sambac absolute, Jasminum grandiflorum* |
| Juniper Berry | *Juniperus communis* |
| Lavender | *Lavandula angustifolia* |
| Lemon | *Citrus x limon* |
| Mandarin | *Citrus reticulata* |
| Neroli | *Citrus x aurantium* |
| Orange, Sweet | *Citrus sinensis* |

| | |
|---|---|
| Peppermint | *Mentha x piperita* |
| Petitgrain | *Citrus aurantium* |
| Pine | *Pinus sylvestris* |
| *Rosalina* | *Melaleuca ericifolia* |
| Rose | *Rosa damascena* |
| Sandalwood | *Santalum album or Santalum spicatum* |
| Spearmint | *Mentha spicata* |
| Tangerine | *Citrus reticulata* |
| Tea Tree | *Melaleuca alternifolia* |

# Essential Oils Safe While Nursing

| | |
|---|---|
| Amyris | *Amyris balsamifera* |
| Balsam Fir | *Abies balsamea* |
| Bergamot | *Citrus bergamia* |
| Black Pepper | *Piper nigrum* |
| Blue Tansy | *Tanacetum annuum* |
| Cedarwood | *Juniperus virginiana* |
| Clary Sage | *Salvia sclarea* |
| Copaiba | *Copaifera langsdofii, Copaifera officinalis* |
| Coriander | *Coriandrum sativum* |
| Cypress | *Cupressus sempervirens* |
| Dill Weed | *Anethum graveolens* |
| Fir Needle | *Abies alba, Abies sachalinensis, Abies sibirica* |
| Fragonia | *Agonis fragrans* |
| Frankincense | *Boswellia carterii* |
| Geranium | *Pelargonium graveolens* |
| Grapefruit | *Citrus paradisi* |
| Helichrysum | *Helichrysum italicum, Helichrysum splendidum* |
| Jasmine | *Jasminum sambac absolute, Jasminum grandiflorum* |
| Juniper Berry | *Juniperus communis* |

| | |
|---|---|
| Lavandin | *Lavandula intermedia* |
| Lavender | *Lavandula angustifolia* |
| Lemon | *Citrus x limon* |
| Lemon Eucalyptus | *Eucalyptus citriodora or Corymbia citriodora* |
| Mandarin | *Citrus reticulata* |
| Marjoram, Sweet | *Origanum majorana* |
| Neroli | *Citrus x aurantium* |
| Orange | *Citrus sinensis* |
| Petitgrain | *Citrus aurantium* |
| Pine | *Pinus sylvestris* |
| *Rosalina* | *Melaleuca ericifolia* |
| Rose | *Rosa damascena* |
| Rosemary | *Rosmarinus officinalis* |
| Sandalwood | *Santalum album or Santalum spicatum* |
| Spearmint | *Mentha spicata* |
| Spruce | *Picea abies* |
| Tangerine | *Citrus reticulata* |
| Tea Tree | *Melaleuca alternifolia* |
| Vetiver | *Vetiveria zizanioides* |

# Essential Oils to Avoid During Pregnancy

| | |
|---|---|
| Aniseed | *Pimpinella anisum* |
| Anise, Star | *Illicium verum* |
| Basil ct. estragole | *Ocimum basilicum* |
| Birch | *Betula lenta* |
| Blue Tansy | *Tanacetum annuum* |
| Camphor | *Cinnamomum camphora* |
| Cassia | *Cinnamomum cassia, Cinnamomum aromaticum* |
| Cinnamon Bark | *Cinnamomum verum, Cinnamomum zeylanicum* |
| Hyssop | *Hyssopus officinalis* |
| Mugwort | *Artemisia vulgaris* |
| Myrrh | *Commiphora myrrha, Commiphora molmol* |
| Oregano | *Origanum vulgare, Origanium onites* |
| Parsley Seed or Leaf | *Petroselinum sativum* |
| Pennyroyal | *Mentha pulegium* |
| Ravintsara (Ho Leaf ct Camphor) | *Cinnamomum camphora* |
| Sage | *Salvia officinalis* |
| Tansy | *Tanacetum vulgare* |
| Tarragon | *Artemisia dracunculus* |

| Thuja | *Thuja occidentalis* |
| Wintergreen | *Gaultheria procumbens* |
| Wormwood | *Artemisia absinthium* |

Other oils that may be questionable or considered too harsh to use during pregnancy include Clove, Davana, Lemongrass, Linden Blossom, Oakmoss, Palo Santo, and Ravensara.

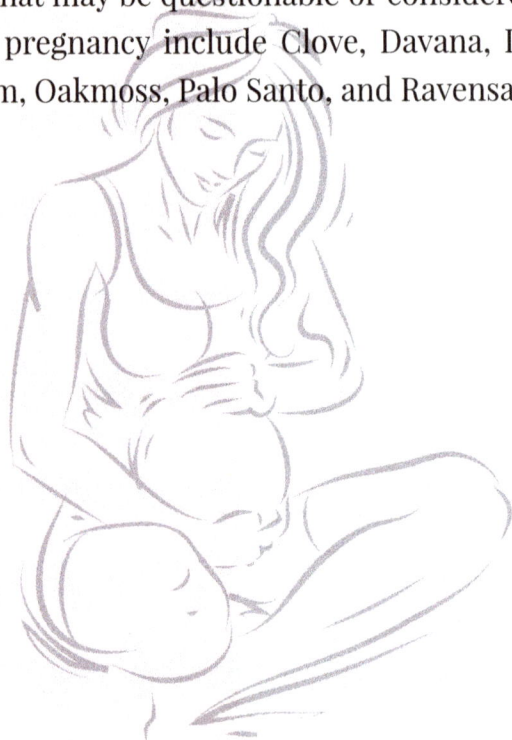

# Baby Safe Essential Oils 3+ Months

The following are the gentlest essential oils considered safe to use on babies three months and older. You will want to first test and watch for any sensitivities. Begin with one essential oil (only one per day) in a tiny amount, then watch very closely for any signs of allergic reactions. Wait 24 hours before trying a different oil. A highly allergic reaction will occur within 15-20 minutes after inhalation or topical application. A mild reaction will occur within 24 hours after introduction to the oil (typically dermal). The dilution rate for this age is 0.1 percent or one drop of essential oil per one ounce of carrier oil for topical applications.

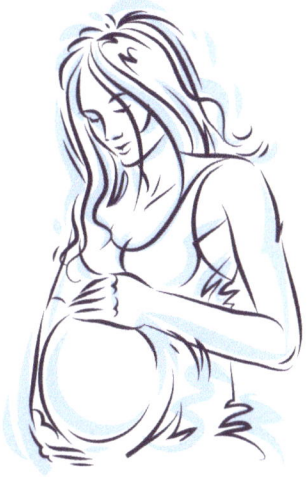

| Lavender | *Lavandula angustifolia* |
| Mandarin | *Citrus reticulata* |
| Orange | *Citrus sinensis* |
| Tangerine | *Citrus reticulata* |
| German Chamomile | *Chamomilla recutita* |
| Roman Chamomile | *Chamaemelum nobile* |
| Rosalina | *Melaleuca ericifolia* |

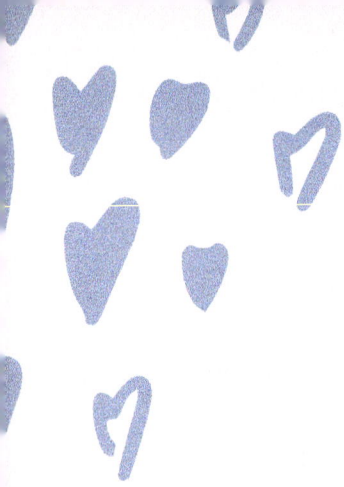

# Therapeutic Properties
# of Essential Oils

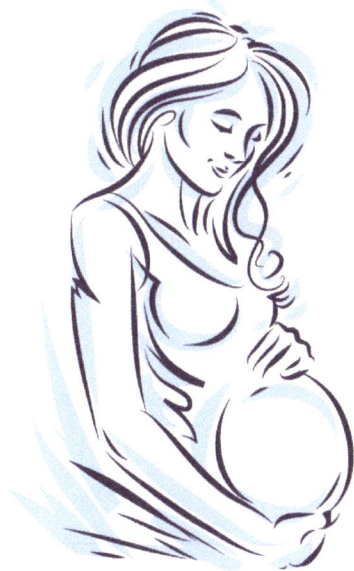

Essential oils contain a complex amalgamation of natural compounds which determines their fragrance and therapeutic properties. Like all other living matter, essential oils contain chemical compounds made up of oxygen, carbon, and hydrogen which together create a synergy of different constituents that endow them with antibacterial, antiviral, antifungal, and antiseptic properties.

Remember, it's the therapeutic actions and the chemistry of an oil that determines which oil is appropriate for use in pregnancy.

Essential oil compounds may be categorized into two distinct chemical groups: hydrocarbons, which are made up of terpenes (monoterpenes, sesquiterpenes, diterpenes, and triterpenes) and oxygenated compounds, which includes esters, aldehydes, ketones, alcohols, phenols, and oxides.

## Monoterpenes

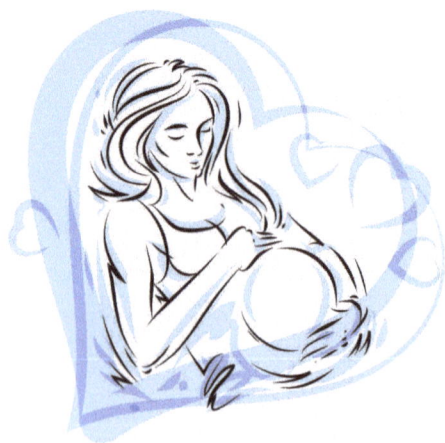

Monoterpenes are a part of almost every essential oil. Around 90% of citrus oils contain limonene, which has the ability to kill viruses. Although potential skin irritants, monoterpenes have many positive abilities—they are generally antibacterial and antiseptic, with stimulating, expectorant, and decongestant properties.

Essential Oils High in Monoterpenes: black pepper, frankincense, atlas cedarwood, bergamot, lemon, grapefruit, cypress, juniper berry, niaouli, and rosemary

## Sesquiterpenes

Sesquiterpenes are generally calming, cooling, antiseptic, antibacterial, analgesic, anti-inflammatory, with sedative and antispasmodic properties. With a unique ability to cross the blood-brain barrier, they can increase the oxygen level of brain tissue and stimulate the pineal and pituitary glands.

Essential Oils High in Sesquiterpenes: cedarwood, ginger, sandalwood, patchouli, and vetiver

## Alcohols

Alcohols are usually non-toxic and not known to cause skin irritation, despite being highly germicidal against bacteria, viruses, and fungi. With a pleasant, uplifting fragrance, they are considered to be extremely therapeutic in aromatherapy. They also provide antiviral, antifungal, and antibacterial properties.

Essential Oils High in Alcohols: clary sage, citronella, geranium, lavender, rose, and tea tree

## Aldehydes

Known for their citrus-like—and sometimes aphrodisiac—fragrances, aldehydes are generally calming and a sedative to the nervous system. Oils high in aldehydes have a robust aroma typically with anti-inflammatory, antiviral, and hypotensive qualities. It's important to properly dilute essential oils high in aldehydes because they can be irritating to the skin when misused.

Essential Oils High in Aldehydes: citronella, eucalyptus citriodora, lemongrass, and melissa (lemon balm)

## Ketones

Although ketones can be toxic in high doses, they offer therapeutic benefits when used with care during pregnancy. Ketones are known for their expectorant and decongestant properties that help the flow of mucus from the body. With analgesic properties, they can be calming and sedative, helping to reduce pain, aid digestion, reduce inflammation, improve scar healing, and regenerate new tissue.

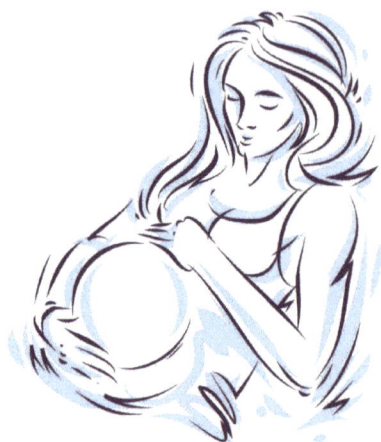

Essential Oils High in Ketones: eucalyptus globulus, rosemary verbena, eucalyptus dives, jasmine, hyssop, camphor, and sage

## Esters

Most plant acids are water-soluble, so they are not abundant in steam-distilled essential oils but instead are more commonly found in hydrosols. Esters are not usually the main component of an essential oil—however, even in minute amounts, they play a vital role in the fruity note of their fragrance. They are also antifungal, anti-inflammatory, antispasmodic, sedative, and calming to the skin and nervous system. They are very gentle in their actions and are the most friendly of all the groups.

Essential Oils High in Esters: lavender, clary sage, geranium, petitgrain, Roman chamomile, bergamot

## Phenols

Phenols are known to be powerful, so they should only be used in a low concentration for a short period. Highly antiseptic, phenols are effective at both killing and preventing the growth of bacteria, fungi, and viruses. They can also stimulate the immune system and aid depression. Due to their strength, phenols can be highly irritating to the skin and may cause liver toxicity with long-term use. Thyme and oregano are known as 'hot oils' due to the burning sensation they can produce on the skin. Oils in this group should be avoided in pregnancy and while breastfeeding.

Essential Oils High in Phenols: clove, cinnamon, oregano, and mountain savory

## Oxides

Oxides can aid the respiratory system due to their expectorant properties—a common example is cineol, which is the main component of eucalyptus oil. They may also have diuretic, antiseptic, and immune-stimulating actions. The most common molecule is 1, 8-cineole, known as eucalyptol. Oxides are commonly found in essential oils from plants in the Myrtaceae family.

Essential Oils High in Oxides: eucalyptus, hyssop, rosemary, and tea tree

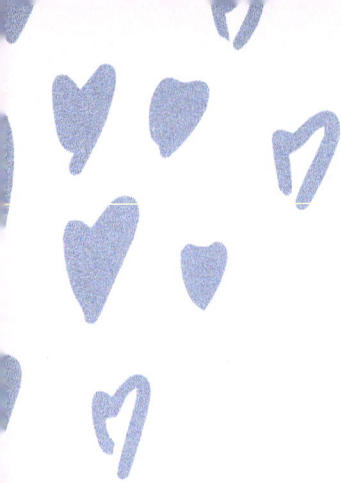

# Chemical Constituents

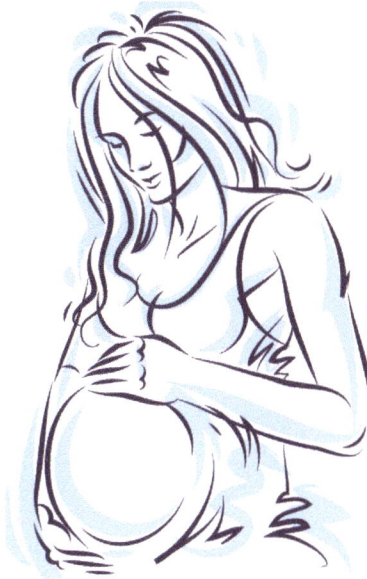

E sters are the most relaxing of the chemical families, and phenols are the most stimulating. Esters are generally considered to have excellent anti-inflammatory, fungicidal, and (cicatrisant) wound-healing properties. Phenols, on the other hand, are excellent antiseptic and bacterial properties but could cause skin irritation. This chart shows each main chemical family and its effect on the nervous system, starting with the gentlest to the most stimulating.

| | |
|---|---|
| Esters | Relaxing |
| Aldehydes | Relaxing |
| Ketones | Relaxing |
| Sesquiterpenes | Balancing |
| Lactones and Coumarins | Balancing |
| Aldehydes (aromatic) | Mildly Stimulating |
| Oxides | Mildly Stimulating |
| Acids | Mildly Stimulating |
| Monoterpenes | Stimulating |
| Alcohols | Stimulating |
| Phenols | Stimulating |

# Things to Consider When Choosing an Oil

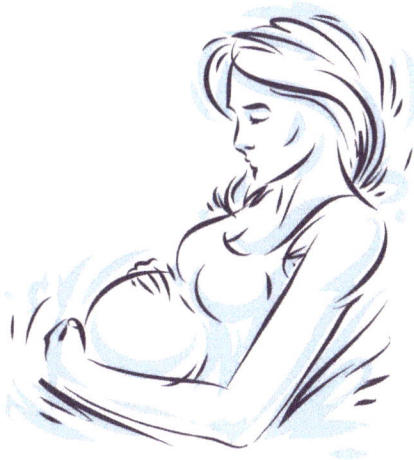

Below are five rules of thumb for using aromatics, especially during this important time in your life.

- Right Oil – Is the oil you're planning to use the right one for the concern that needs to be addressed?

- Right Route – Are you using the oil in the most effective and safest manner possible?

- Right Dose – Are your dilution calculations correct?

- Right Frequency – Are you using the oil frequently enough? What about too often?

- Right Symptom – Are you treating the correct symptom with your remedy? Also, are you addressing both physical needs and emotional ones?

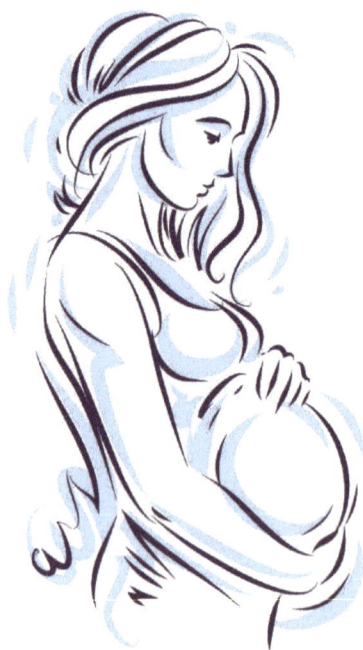

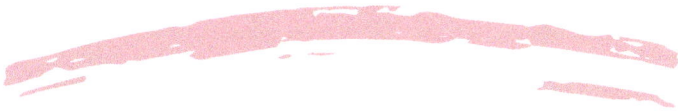

# Carrier Oils

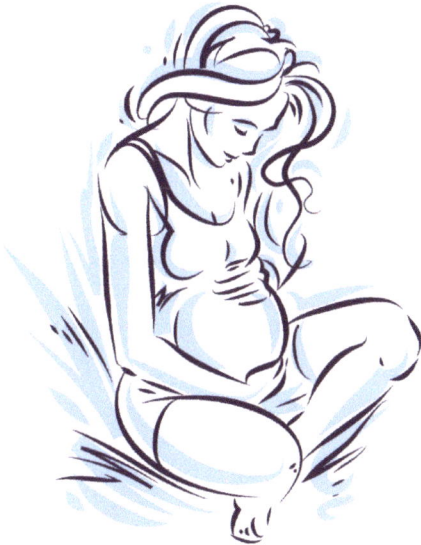

I t is crucial always to dilute essential oils with a carrier before using topically. With the wide selection of carrier oils, each with various therapeutic benefits, choosing one will depend on the area being applied to, the treatment plan, and any skin sensitivities. The list below is a short directory of carrier oils beneficial for making blends during pregnancy and beyond.

## Sweet almond

**Sweet almond** oil is one of the most useful, practical, and moderately priced carrier oils available. It is great for all skin types as it moisturizes and reconditions the skin with its satiny smooth texture. This pale yellow oil quickly absorbs into the skin, leaving your skin feeling soft and non-greasy. Sweet almond provides relief from itching, soreness, dryness, inflammation and is especially beneficial for eczema. As a lightly nutty refined oil rich in fatty acids, proteins, and Vitamin D, it is everyone's favorite massage oil base for loosening stiff muscles and achy joints.

**Dilution:** Can be used at 100%.

## Avocado

**Avocado** oil is rich in lecithin and vitamins A, B1, B2, D, and E. It also contains amino acids, sterols, and pantothenic acid. It is known to delay aging as it is rich in essential fatty acids. Avocado easily penetrates the skin, acts as a sunscreen, and helps in cell regeneration. For skin that has been exposed to the sun, mix zinc oxide in a half bottle of avocado oil and apply. Avocado is greatly praised for those who suffer from skin problems such as eczema, psoriasis, and other skin disorders. For an intensive facial treatment for mature skin, refined avocado oil is preferred as it lacks odor. It is beneficial for dry skin and suitable for all skin types.

**Dilution:** Can be used at 100%, although in most cases, it is best mixed with another carrier oil such as sweet almond or grapeseed oil to make up a 10-30% dilution of the carrier blend.

## Grapeseed

**Grapeseed** oil is a pleasing light green odorless oil, useful as a base oil for many creams, lotions and as a carrier oil. It is especially beneficial for all skin types because of its natural non-allergenic properties. Grapeseed works well, especially when other oils do not absorb well, without leaving a greasy feeling after application. Slightly astringent, it tightens and tones the skin and alleviates acne. Grapeseed makes an ideal carrier oil for body massage bases. Saturation takes longer than some other carrier oils. Suitable for skin sensitivities or allergies.

**Dilution:** Can be used at 100%.

## Jojoba

**Jojoba** oil is bright and golden in color and is known as one of the best oils (really a liquid wax) for hair and skin. It penetrates the skin quickly and is excellent for skin nourishment and for healing inflamed skin, psoriasis, eczema, or any sort of dermatitis. Jojoba controls acne, oily skin and makes a terrific scalp cleanser as excess sebum dissolves in jojoba. It's good for all skin types and promotes a healthy, glowing complexion by gently unclogging the pores and lifting embedded impurities. It makes an excellent base oil for treating rheumatism and arthritis because of its anti-inflammatory actions. Jojoba is suitable for all aromatherapy uses other than a full-body massage. And, because of the oil's antioxidants, it does not become rancid and can even prevent rancidity in other oils with an unlimited shelf life.

**Dilution:** Can be used at 100% but due to its price, many use at a 10% dilution with other carrier oils.

## Coconut

**Coconut** (fractionated) seems to be quickly becoming the carrier oil of choice because of its vast use in alternative medicine and healing. While it is fractionated, no change has been made chemically. Instead, its molecular structure 'fraction' has been separated, allowing it to remain liquid at room temperature, making it much more useful in aromatherapy. Coconut oil is perfect as a moisturizer for the body and conditions brittle, dry, or dull hair. Its light, easily absorbable texture gives skin a smooth satin effect with virtually no scent of its own and indefinite shelf life.

**Dilution:** Can be used at 100%.

## Coconut oil

**Coconut oil** (virgin) has an unbelievable balance of natural saturated fatty acids with antibacterial and antiviral properties not found in other oils. Coconut oil is perfect as a skin conditioner for nearly all skin conditions and is believed to stimulate hair growth. It has a light, aromatic coconut scent and becomes solid at room temperature. For this reason, it is recommended to blend with other carrier oils in your body care products. It is fully digestible and is considered a healthy cooking oil.

**Dilution:** Can be used alone, but it is recommended to use at a 10-25% dilution with other carrier oils.

# Calendula

**Calendula** oil is an infused oil from the petals of marigolds steeped in a pure vegetable oil such as olive or almond oil. It is suitable for all skin types and is valuable for treating wounds, scars, burns, inflammation, and other injuries as it aids in tissue regeneration. Calendula oil contains natural steroid material called sterols and is especially useful for treating skin conditions like eczema or skin damaged by steroid abuse. A 50/50 mixture of calendula oil and St. John's wort oil is an especially effective remedy for the repairing of scarred or damaged skin from burns. It has anti-inflammatory and antispasmodic properties. Due to its vitamin content, calendula works well in moisturizers.

**Dilution:** Use at a 10-25% dilution with another carrier oil or carrier oil blend.

# Cocoa Butter

**Cocoa Butter** is a rich and creamy butter (not a carrier oil) that must be warmed to make it liquid. It is a wonderful addition to skincare products due to its high level of polyphenols, vitamins, and nutrients. It smoothes, hydrates, and balances skin while providing collagen to support mature skin and helps with stretch marks. Its warm aroma of cocoa is a delightful addition in lotions and creams.

**Dilution:** Its solid texture makes it difficult to work it and needs to be blended with other oils to be workable. Use at a

10% dilution.

Other carriers such as Epsom salts and dead sea salts can help alleviate muscle pain and tension, as well as help to add magnesium to the body through dermal absorption. Aloe vera gel can be used for delivering essential oils to targeted areas.

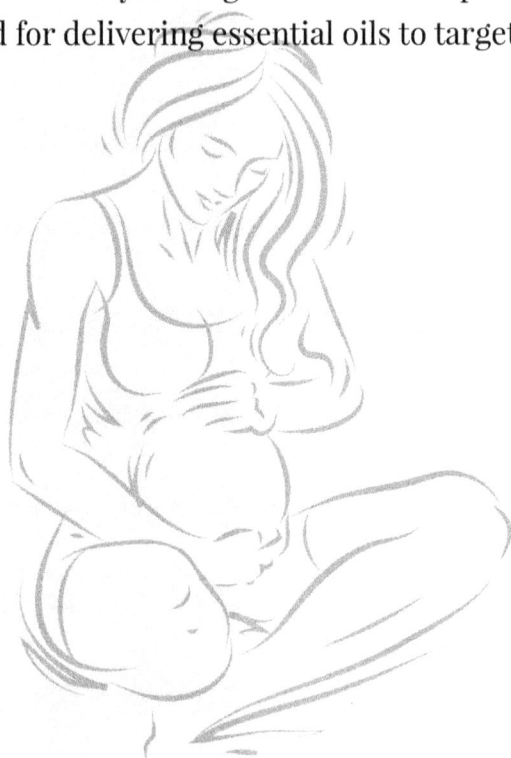

# Hydrosols

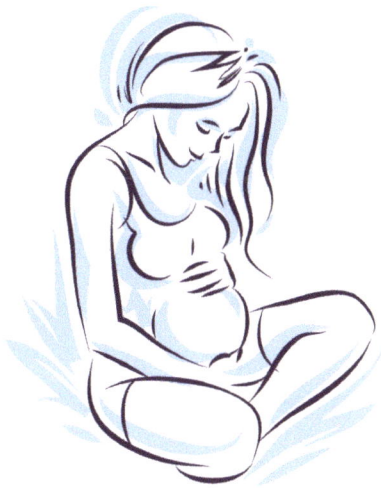

Hydrosols are the by-product of steam distilling essential oils. Although they are considered a by-product, they have many applications in aromatherapy and are especially great for use with infants. Hydrosols contain minute amounts of the actual essential oil, making them much safer and gentler on babies' delicate skin. They are also great as a perineal spray for mom during postpartum. Below is a list of hydrosols that are useful in pregnancy, postpartum, and infant care.

| | |
|---|---|
| **Helichrysum** | Very useful in postpartum care, especially if mom has had an episiotomy. |
| **Lavender** | Calming for mom and baby, useful on diaper rash and skin irritations, as well as for perineal care. |
| **Roman Chamomile** | Calming to mom and baby; helps promote sleep in baby, and great for diaper rash. |
| **Rose** | Helpful for mom with postpartum skin and hair issues, and is very calming and relaxing. |
| **Tea Tree** | Great for perineal care with cleansing properties and keeps infection at bay. |

# Suggested Uses for Aromatherapy During Pregnancy

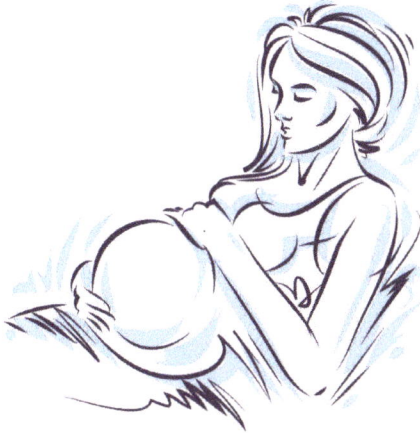

Some of the ways you can use aromatherapy during your pregnancy include a soothing massage, a warm bath, a compress, or by inhalation, to name a few.

- For restful sleep and/or to prevent insomnia, try diffusing lavender essential oil. It helps you to feel calmer and relax more, especially near the end of your pregnancy. Or, create a pillow spray using 12 drops (total) of lavender, ylang ylang, mandarin, and frankincense. Fill the remaining 2-ounce spray bottle with distilled water. Use on the pillow before bedtime.

- If your skin becomes sensitive to touch, try adding essential oils to a warm bath or in a footbath instead.

- To help relieve stress and deal with moodiness, add three drops of lavender essential oil to a carrier oil and massage into your upper back and neck. Other favorite essential oils can be used as well to help in lifting your mood.

- Lavender can help relieve headaches. For emotional stress, add a couple of drops of lavender with a carrier oil into the palm of your hand and blend. Rub into wrists, neck, and around ears.

- For high blood pressure during pregnancy, mix three drops of ylang ylang essential oil into two tablespoons of

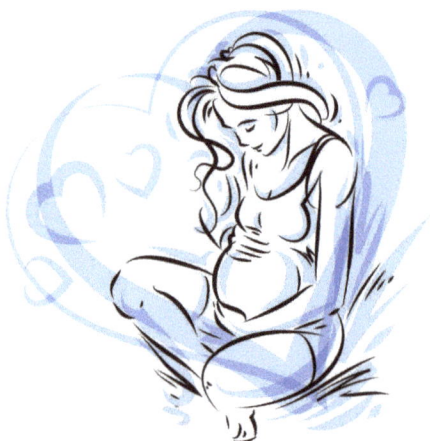

dead sea salts for a relaxing bath.

- Using black pepper essential oil helps relieve various aches and pains during pregnancy.

- For muscle aches, try lavender, ylang ylang, ginger, frankincense, and chamomile. Add a total of 12 drops of essential oil to two tablespoons of a carrier oil such as almond oil.

- Peppermint and spearmint oil help relieve morning sickness during the first trimester of pregnancy. You can also diffuse three drops of grapefruit essential oil by your bed in the morning to stave off nausea.

- To avoid stretch marks, blend two drops of helichrysum, four drops of lavender, one drop of frankincense and five drops of bergamot to a tablespoon of rosehip and hazelnut oil blend and massage on location a couple of times a day.

- For gas (flatulence) or bloating, place one drop of peppermint on the tongue.

- Tangerine essential oil helps relieve fatigue and tiredness.

- For swelling and water retention, add a drop or two of lemon essential oil to drinking water daily. To make a blend for edema around the ankles, add three drops of geranium, ginger, lemon, and lavender to a 10 ml bottle of fractionated coconut oil. Massage into feet and ankles, rubbing upward toward the heart.

- Tea tree oil helps prevent and relieve symptoms of a cold. Add a few drops to a diffuser when congested. Myrtle also helps relieve nasal congestion.

- For yeast infections, blend three drops of tea tree essential oil with one drop of lavender into two tablespoons of dead sea salts. Add to running warm bath water. Soak for ten minutes.

- Tangerine and lavender essential oils are helpful for mastitis (infected breasts).

- For hemorrhoids, use a local compress of essential oils with cypress, frankincense, and lavender to soothe and heal. These oils can also be added to your daily bath. Or, you can mix eight drops (total) tea tree, cypress, geranium, and lavender to two tablespoons of aloe vera gel and apply to the affected area with a tissue.

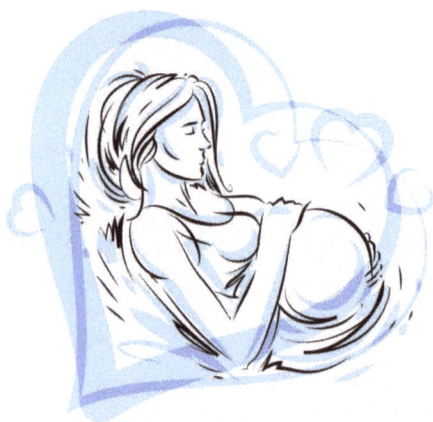

- For lower back and leg pain, add a few drops of geranium with a carrier oil on location.

- Essential oils used for labor pain and childbirth include cinnamon leaf, jasmine, lavender, nutmeg, parsley, rose, and clary sage. Place two drops of essential oil into one tablespoon of carrier oil and massage into hips, abdomen, and soles of the feet. Or, use a warm compress with two drops of ylang ylang or lavender essential oil on the abdomen or back.

- Essential oils helpful with lactation and lack of nursing milk include basil, celery seed, clary sage, dill, fennel, and hops. Massage five drops of essential oils with one tablespoon carrier oil into breasts and upper chest. Wash nipple area thoroughly before nursing.

- For nipple soreness, use helichrysum or lavender essential oil to soothe and heal faster. Lavender is also beneficial for engorgement. Add two drops of lavender and two drops of geranium to a warm compress to lay across the chest for comfort. Be sure to thoroughly clean essential oils off before nursing.

- To avoid dried or cracked nipples, add a blend of geranium, lavender, and sandalwood essential oils to a tablespoon of carrier oil and gently massage in. Be sure to wash the nipple area thoroughly before nursing.

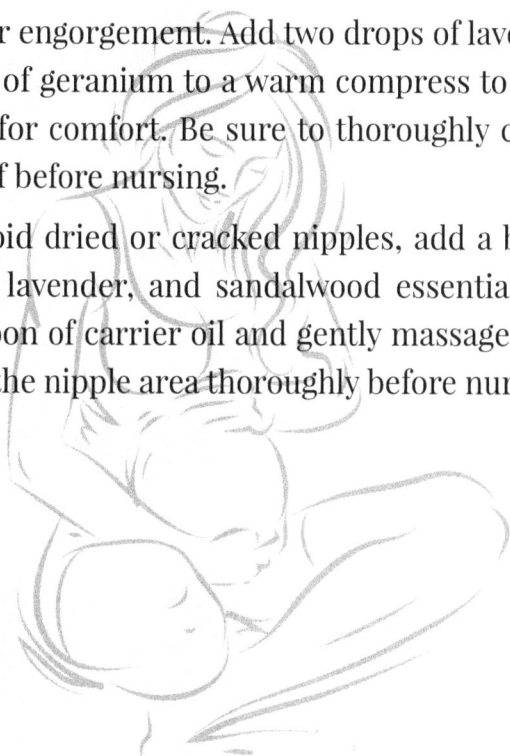

# Pregnancy – The Journey

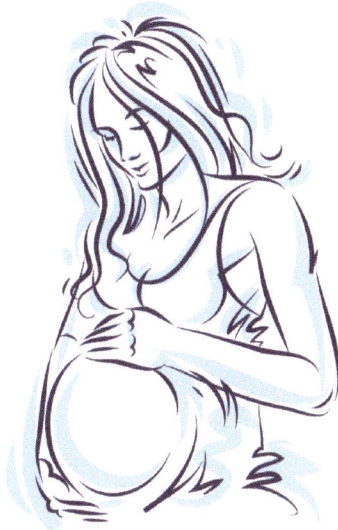

Essential oils provide support to the mother-to-be in alleviating unpleasant symptoms that may arise during pregnancy, labor, and delivery. In this chapter, we will be looking at some of the common causes of discomfort during pregnancy such as anemia, constipation, genital infections, hemorrhoids, high or low blood pressure, nausea and vomiting, urinary tract infections, heartburn, and moodiness and how essential oils can bring relief. Please note, some complications of pregnancy will need medical intervention such as high blood pressure, gestational diabetes, iron-deficiency anemia, and severe nausea and vomiting, among others.

## Acne

Hormones associated with pregnancy can wreak havoc on the mom's skin and cause acne that can be similar in severity to teenage acne. Acne during pregnancy occurs when your hair follicles become plugged with oil and dead skin cells. It often causes whiteheads, blackheads or pimples, and usually appears on the face, forehead, chest, upper back and shoulders. Depending on its severity, using essential oils can minimize scarring and heal acne quickly.

When using essential oils for acne, topically is the route you want to go with—a nice facial moisturizer, salve, serum, or spot-treatment roller bottle are all great ideas. Essential oils that can help with this include bergamot, geranium, lavender, lemon, lime, mandarin, neroli, niaouli, palmarosa, petitgrain, rose, sandalwood, and tea tree.

## Acne Spot Treatment Salve

**What You Will Need:**

1 ½ ounce (3 teaspoons) apricot oil
1 teaspoon beeswax
3 drops lime essential oil
3 drops neroli essential oil
3 drops rose essential oil
3 drops geranium essential oil
2-ounce tin container
small saucepan

**What To Do:**

1.  In a small saucepan over very low heat, combine the apricot oil and beeswax.

2.  Once the beeswax has melted, add the essential oils and stir gently to combine.

3.  Pour the liquid into a two-ounce stainless steel tin and allow it to cool completely before replacing the lid. Add a label so you don't forget what it is!

**To Use:** After washing your face, dab a small amount of this salve over the affected areas (a little goes a long way). It may take some time to be absorbed, so this is best done before bed. When you wake up, your skin will be beautifully soft and oil-free.

## Zit Zapper Salve

**What You Will Need:**

2 tablespoons beeswax beads
2 tablespoons shea butter
1 tablespoon coconut oil
6 drops tea tree essential oil
6 drops lavender essential oil
3 drops palmarosa essential oil
3 drops rosemary essential oil

**What To Do:**

1. Melt the beeswax, shea butter, and coconut oil together in a glass jar in a simmering saucepan of water.

2. Once melted, add your essential oils and mix quickly.

3. Pour the mixture into lip balm containers or craft tubes for ease of use. Allow to cool and set. Make up a few to have on hand at home, school, or work.

**To Use:** Dab a small amount directly on the pimple when it appears.

# Anxiety

Hormonal changes or even thinking about the upcoming labor or birth of the baby can all cause the mom-to-be to have some anxious feelings. Anxiety is a feeling of unease, such as worry or fear that can be mild or severe. Its perfectly normal to have feelings of anxiety during your pregnancy—for example, how the delivery will go and caring for the new addition in the home. Use essential oils to ease your worries and quiet your mind.

Aromatic use is the method of choice for anxiety, such as diffusion or personal inhalers. Essential oils that can help with this include bergamot, Virginian cedarwood, Roman chamomile, frankincense, jasmine, lavender, lemon, lime, marjoram, neroli, palmarosa, patchouli, rose, sandalwood, vetiver, ylang ylang, and orange.

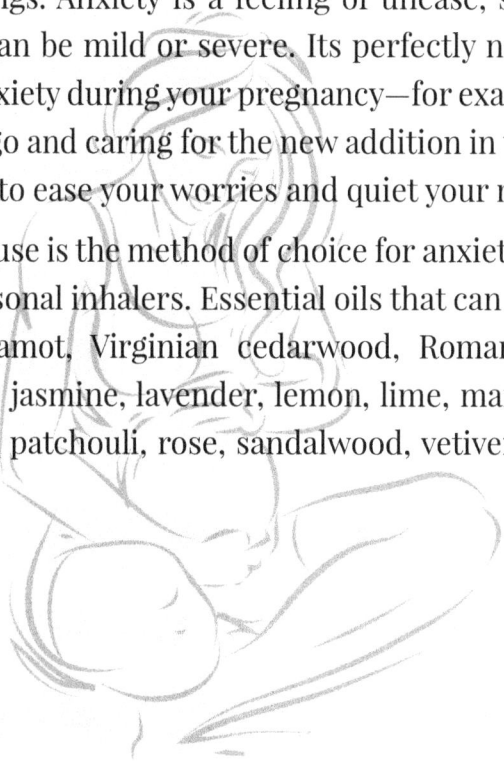

## Anxiety Diffuser Blend

**What You Will Need:**

2 drops frankincense essential oil
2 drops neroli essential oil
1 drop patchouli essential oil
1 drop ylang ylang essential oil
15 ml size glass bottle

**What To Do:**

1. Add each essential oil to an ultrasonic water diffuser and run as usual. If using a cool-air nebulizing diffuser, multiply this blend by 10 and place in a 15 ml glass bottle and run for 30 minutes to one hour before going to bed.

2. Or, if no diffuser is available, place one to two drops of the blend to palms and take three to five deep breaths.

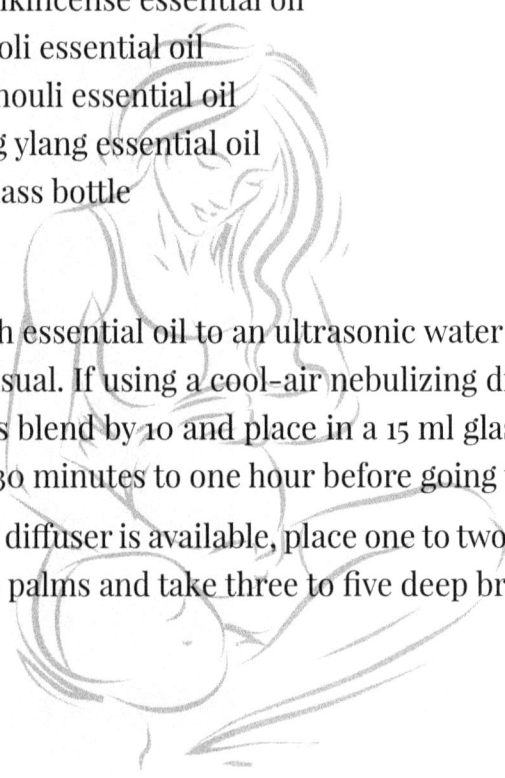

## *Take It Easy Personal Inhaler*

**What You Will Need:**

> 5 drops jasmine essential oil (or substitute: ylang ylang)
> 5 drops lavender essential oil
> 5 drop bergamot essential oil
> 1 plastic inhaler
> small bowl

**What To Do:**

1. In a small glass bowl, add the essential oils. Stir to blend.

2. Place the white cotton wick in the bowl using your tweezers and soak it in the oils. Roll it around, allowing the cotton to soak up all the oil.

3. Place the cotton in the bottom of the inhaler tube and seal the tube securely with the "butt" of the inhaler. Replace cap to cover opening and prevent it from drying out.

**To Use:** Inhale several times daily as needed (3–5 times a day in general).

## Anti-Anxiety Roller Blend

**What You Will Need:**

1 teaspoon fractionated coconut oil
2 drops cedarwood essential oil
2 drops orange essential oil
1 drop ylang ylang essential oil
1 drop patchouli essential oil
1-5 ml glass roll-on bottle
pipette

**What To Do:**

1. Remove the rollerball and add the carrier oil, leaving a little space at the top for essential oils.

2. Add essential oils—it is best to use two to three oils to create a synergy blend.

3. Fill the rest of the space with a carrier oil, then replace roller ball and lid.

4. Use as needed on wrists, temples, and back of the neck.

# Backache

During a pregnancy, nagging backaches can occur due to the extra weight the mom-to-be is carrying or pressure on an old injury. Backaches are best treated through topical use—massage oil, bath salts, or a spray liniment would all be good choices. Essential oils that can help with this include black pepper, eucalyptus, ginger, lavender, lemon, peppermint, and pine.

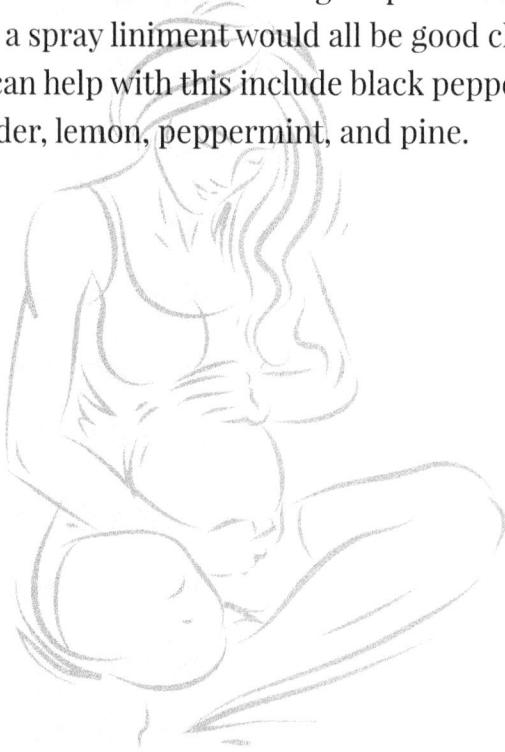

## Back Pain Massage Oil

**What You Will Need:**

1-ounce plastic or glass squeeze-top bottle
1-ounce coconut oil (or another carrier oil)
1 drop black pepper essential oil
2 drops peppermint essential oil
3 drops lavender essential oil

**What To Do:**

1. Place all of your essential oils into an empty squeeze-top bottle.

2. Top the bottle off with the carrier oil of your choice.

3. Replace the cap and shake the bottle to mix.

**To Use**: Massage into the lower back to help relieve pain.

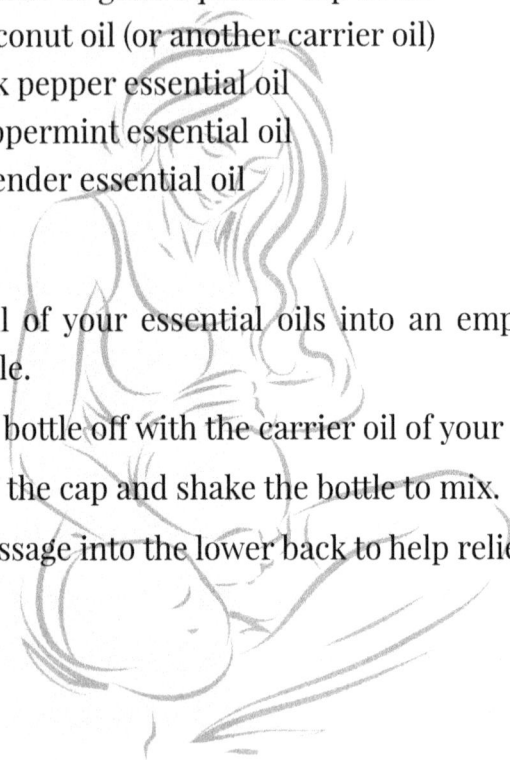

## *Back Pain Relief Balm*

**What You Will Need:**

½ tablespoon castor oil
½ tablespoon tamanu oil
½ ounce beeswax
3 ½ ounces olive oil (infused with arnica, comfrey, and dandelion flower)
6 drops peppermint essential oil
4 drops ginger essential oil
2 drops eucalyptus essential oil
glass jar

**What To Do:**

1. In a glass jar, add castor oil, tamanu oil, beeswax, and infused olive oil.

2. Set the heatproof jar in a small saucepan containing an inch or two of water. Place the pan over a medium-low burner and heat until the beeswax is melted.

3. Remove from heat, cool slightly, then stir in essential oils.

4. Pour mixture into small tins or jars. This recipe yields four ounces of balm.

**To Use**: Massage into the lower back to help relieve pain.

# Breast Tenderness

An increase in size or hormones can both cause the pregnant woman's breast to feel sore—topical use of essential oils is the preferred method of delivery. Breast pain, also known as mastalgia, mammalgia, and mastodynia, is common and may include a dull ache, heaviness, tightness, a burning sensation in the breast tissue, or breast tenderness. Try making a nice, nourishing cream or massage oil. Essential oils that can help with this include black pepper, cypress, lavender, frankincense, German or Roman chamomile, helichrysum, marjoram, rosalina, geranium, and ylang ylang.

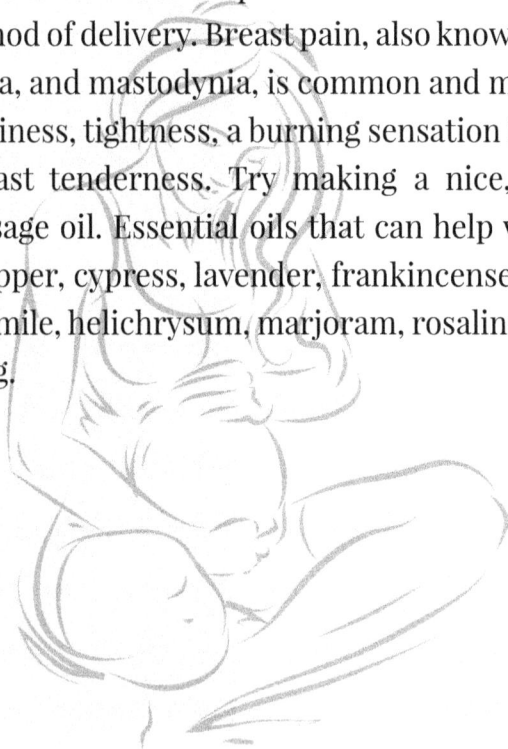

## *Boob Roller Balm*

**What You Will Need:**

> 1-ounce fractionated coconut oil (or substitute: tamanu oil)
> 3 drops lavender essential oil
> 5 drops frankincense essential oil
> 4 drops German chamomile essential oil

**What To Do:**

1. In a roll-on bottle, add essential oils. Fill the remaining space with fractionated coconut oil.

2. Replace ball and top and give it a good shake before each use. Apply as needed. Be sure to wash off completing before nursing.

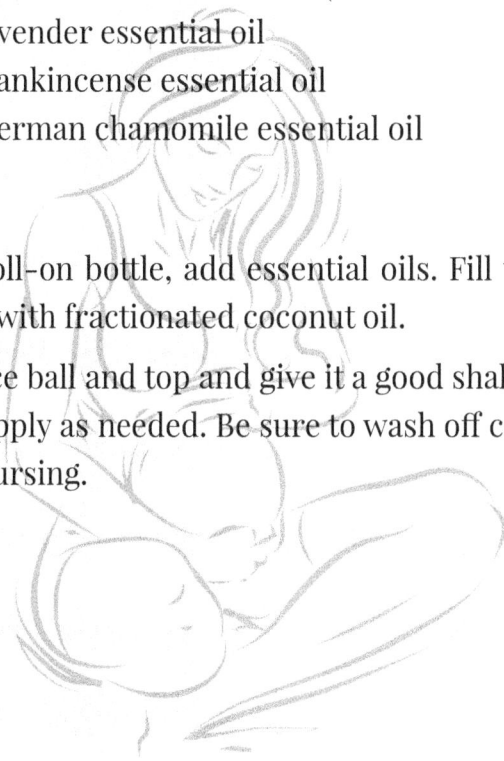

## Soothing Breast Massage Oil

**What You Will Need:**

1-ounce plastic squeeze-top bottle

1-ounce coconut oil (or another carrier oil such as hemp or olive)

1 drop marjoram essential oil

2 drops cypress essential oil

3 drops helichrysum essential oil

**What To Do:**

1. Place all of your essential oils into an empty squeeze-top bottle.

2. Top the bottle off with the carrier oil of your choice.

3. Replace the cap and shake the bottle to mix.

**To Use**: Massage into the breasts as needed. Be sure to wash off thoroughly before nursing baby.

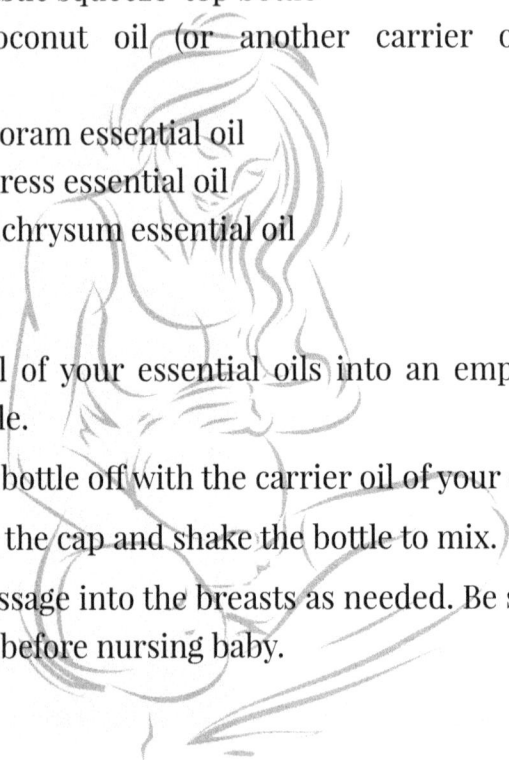

# Constipation

The digestive system changes during pregnancy and generally becomes much slower, which can lead to constipation for mom. Constipation can be treated through topical use, such as a massage oil for the abdomen, or through a rectal suppository. Essential oils that can help include black pepper, ginger, orange, peppermint, pine, and rosemary.

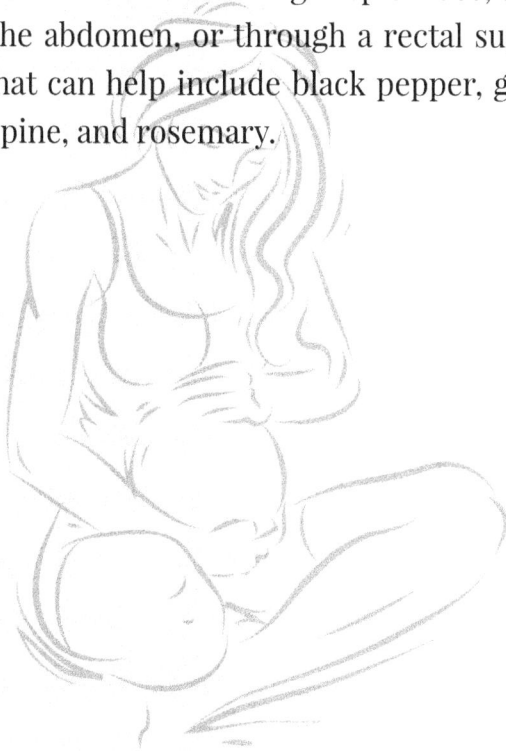

## Belly Bomb Massage Oil

**What You Will Need:**

1-ounce plastic squeeze-top bottle

1-ounce grapeseed oil (or another carrier oil such as almond)

1 drop black pepper essential oil

2 drops peppermint essential oil

3 drops ginger essential oil

**What To Do:**

1. Place all of your essential oils into an empty squeeze-top bottle.

2. Top the bottle off with the carrier oil of your choice.

3. Replace the cap and shake the bottle to mix.

**To Use:** Massage the blend over abdomen in a clockwise direction. Repeat two to three times daily or as needed.

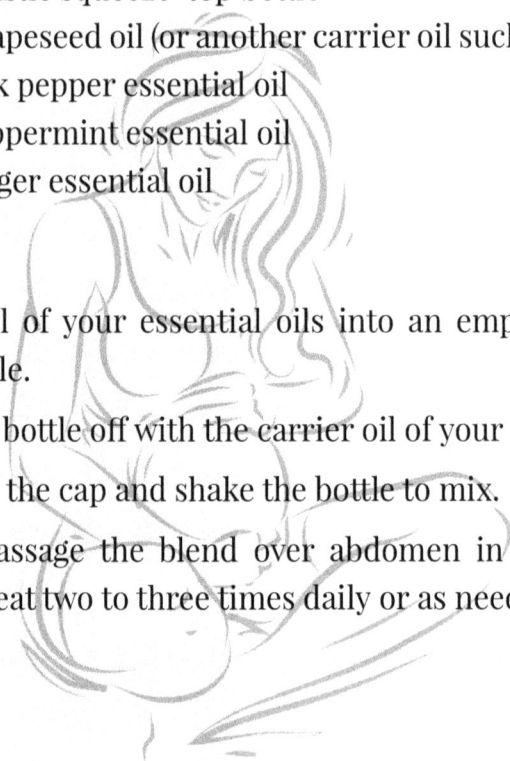

## *Abdominal Massage Oil*

**What You Will Need:**

> 1-ounce plastic squeeze-top bottle
>
> 1-ounce carrier oil (such as argan, almond, or macadamia)
>
> 2 drops peppermint essential oil
>
> 2 drops rosemary essential oil
>
> 2 drops orange essential oil

**What To Do:**

1. Combine carrier oil and essential oils in a plastic bottle.

2. Replace the cap and shake the bottle to mix.

**To Use:** Massage the blend over abdomen in a clockwise direction. Repeat two to three times daily or as needed.

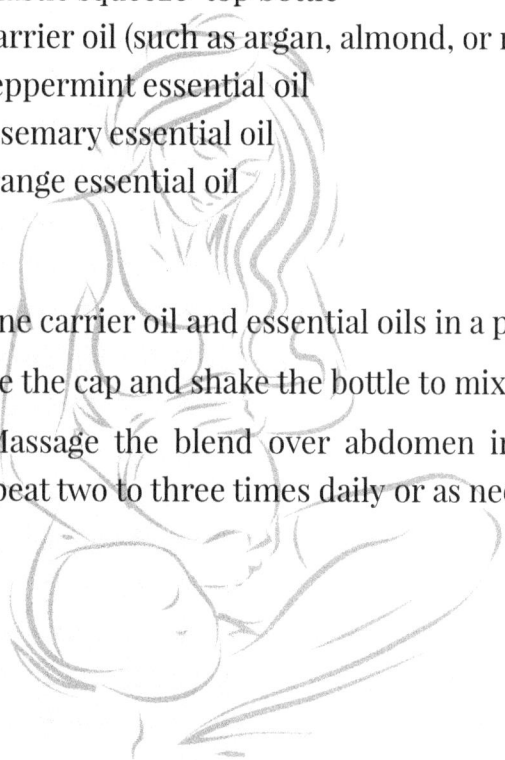

## Constipation Compress

**What You Will Need:**

4 drops rosemary essential oil

2 drops black pepper essential oil

2 drops peppermint essential oil

towel for hot or cold compress

**What To Do:**

1. In a large bowl of hot or cold water, add essential oils.

2. Soak a towel in the water and ring out.

**To Use:** Use towel as a compress on your lower abdomen to get your digestive tract back on track.

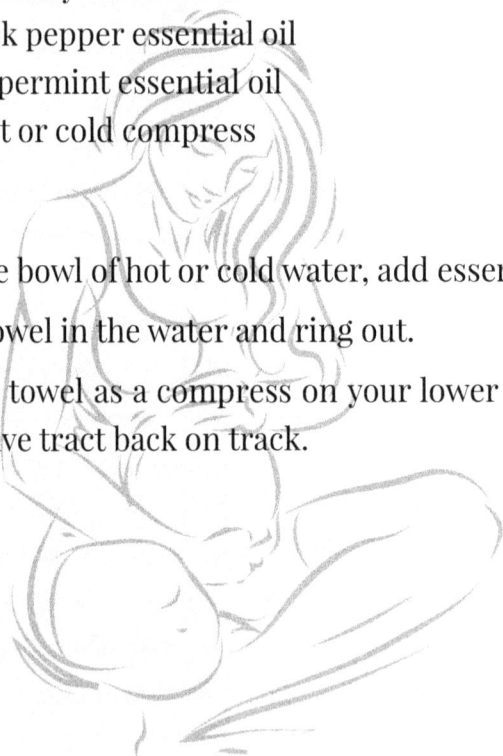

# Depression

Sometimes mom can become depressed throughout her pregnancy, especially if her pregnancy is complicated or has received not-optimal news about her child. Depression is a common medical illness that negatively affects how you feel, the way you think and how you act. Fortunately, it is also treatable. Depression that can cause feelings of sadness can lead to a variety of emotional and physical problems and can decrease a person's ability to function at work and at home.

Depression is also common after delivery in the form of Postpartum Depression. Using essential oils aromatically is the best way to address depression. Essential oils that can help include bergamot, Roman chamomile, frankincense, geranium, jasmine, lavender, lemon, mandarin, may chang, neroli, peppermint, pine, rose, sandalwood, tangerine, and ylang ylang.

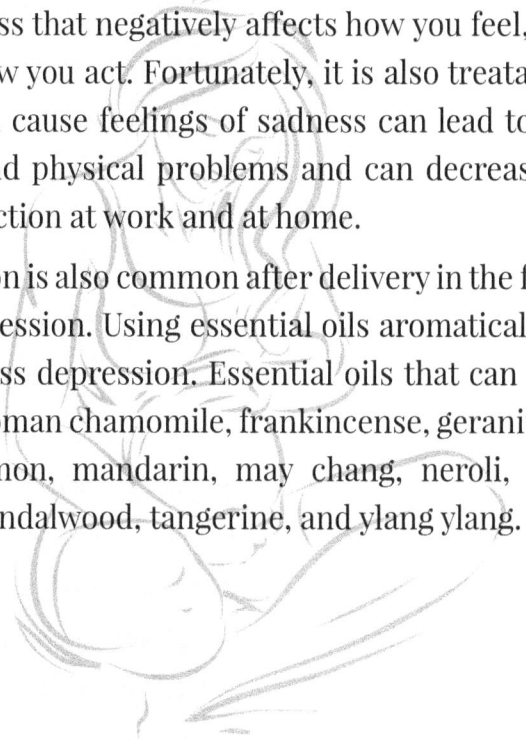

## Joyful Mama Bath Soak

**What You Will Need:**

4 drops Roman chamomile essential oil
4 drops lavender essential oil
2 drops bergamot essential oil
2 drops sandalwood essential oil
2 ounces dead sea salts or pink himalayan salts
plastic tub or container with lid

**What To Do:**

1. In a dark glass bowl, combine the bath salts and essential oils. Mix well.

2. Store in a container, ready for use. Makes 2-4 uses.

**To Use:** Add ½ cup to a running bath. Swish around with your hand to ensure salts dissolve. Soak in water for 15-20 minutes.

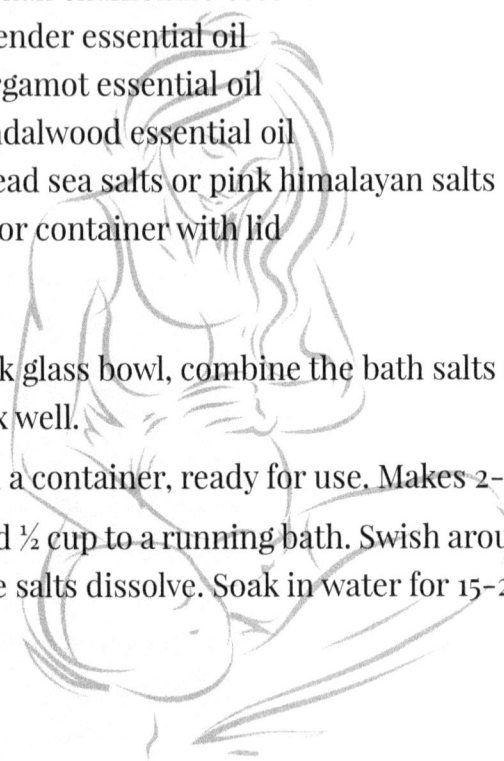

## Momma Time Bath Blend

**What You Will Need:**

1 teaspoon glycerin, gel, or aloe vera
3 drops mandarin essential oil
2 drops pine essential oil
1 drop sandalwood essential oil
small dish or bowl

**What To Do:**

1. In a small dish or bowl, add the glycerin or gel as your fixative.

2. Add your essential oils one drop at a time to the fixative and stir well.

3. Pour your bath blend into a stream of warm running bathwater. Enjoy!

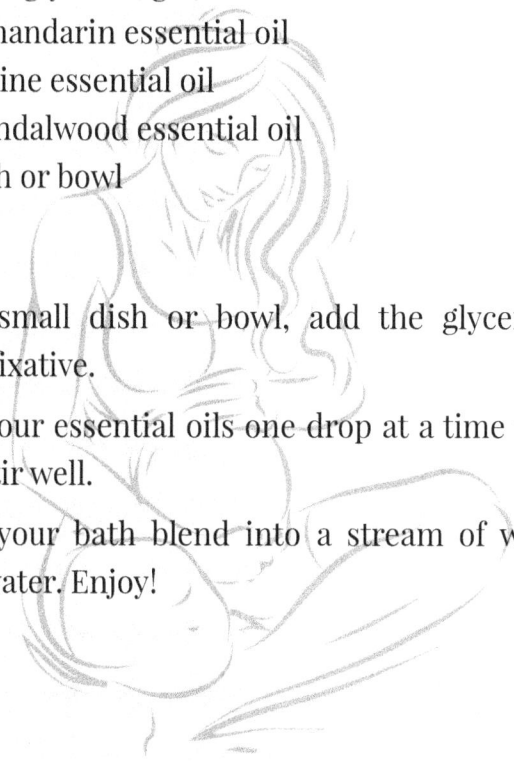

## *Tropical Bath Soak*

**What You Will Need:**

3 drops neroli essential oil
2 drops geranium essential oil
2 drops patchouli essential oil
2 drops ylang ylang essential oil
1 drop bergamot essential oil
1 tablespoon coconut oil
3 cups epsom salts

**What To Do:**

1. Combine all essential oils and coconut oil. Mix well.

2. In a bowl add the epsom or sea salt, using a spoon to mix. Pour the oil blend into the bowl and mix well with the salts.

3. Transfer the bath salt blend in an airtight container and store in a cool, dark place.

**To Use:** Add ½ cup to one cup of salts to running water. Make sure the bath salt blend dissolves completely before getting into the tub. Get in, relax and enjoy!

## *Oh Happy Day Room Spray*

**What You Will Need**

> 2 ounces lavender or neroli hydrosol (or distilled water)
>
> 1 tablespoon glycerin (as a fixative)
>
> 5-7 drops grapefruit essential oil
>
> 4-6 drops lavender essential oil
>
> 3-5 drops chamomile essential oil
>
> glass or plastic spray bottle

**What To Do:**

1. In a clean spray bottle, add the glycerin.

2. Add your essential oils to the fixative. Shake well.

3. Pour the hydrosol or floral water into the bottle and shake to mix contents well.

4. If you want to make this a facial spray instead, use one and a half ounces of hydrosol with one-half ounce of witch hazel.

**To Use:** Spray as needed around your room. If using around children or pets, please check precautions for the essential oils you choose.

# Dizziness

Pregnancy can cause blood pressure fluctuations which can lead to dizziness. Dizziness is a term used to describe a range of sensations, such as feeling faint, woozy, weak, or unsteady. Dizziness that creates the false sense that you or your surroundings are spinning, or moving is called vertigo. Using essential oils via inhalation is the best choice for helping with dizziness. Essential oils that may help include frankincense, peppermint, and pine.

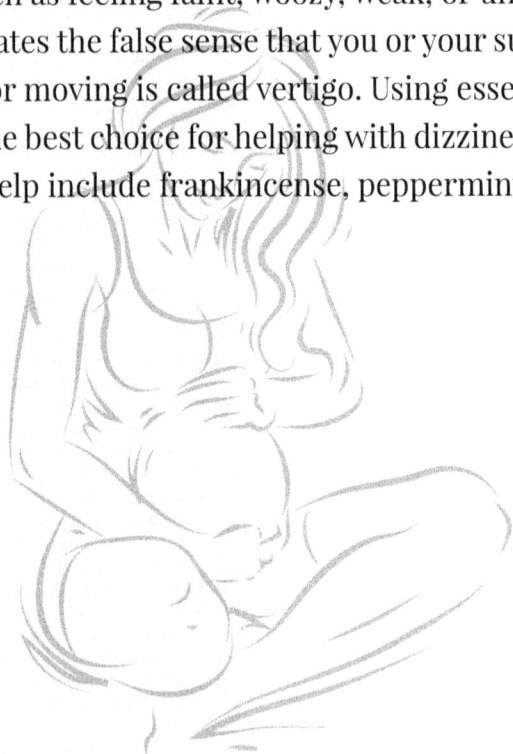

## *Dizzy Tamer*

**What You Will Need:**

2 drops peppermint essential oil
1 drop ginger essential oil
1 drop frankincense essential oil
1 drop rosemary essential oil
2 drops tangerine essential oil
fractionated coconut oil
10 ml roller bottle

**What To Do:**

1. Remove the roller ball from the bottle and add the essential oils drop by drop.

2. Fill the remaining space with fractionated coconut oil.

3. Firmly push the roller ball in, screw on the cap, and shake well to mix the oils.

**To Use:** Roll on the temples, behind ears, and at the base of skull as needed.

## *Woozy Inhaler Blend*

**What You Will Need:**

5 drops peppermint essential oil
3 drops rosemary essential oil
3 drops lavender essential oil
pocket inhaler

**What To Do:**

1. Remove the cotton wick from the inhaler and add the essential oils in a small bowl and stir. Roll wick in the bowl to absorb the oils.

2. Using tweezers, place the wick back inside the inhaler and snap the plug on its bottom.

**To Use:** Take deep breaths from the inhaler as needed.

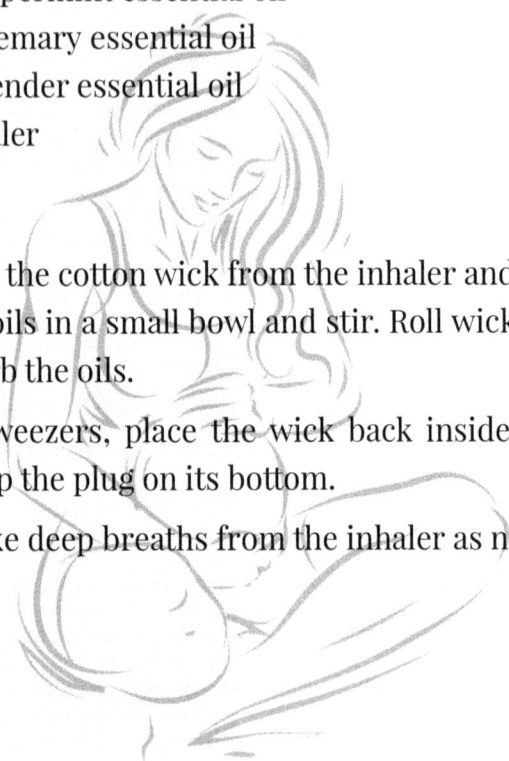

# Edema and Swelling

Water retention can happen at any time and is very prevalent in pregnancy. The swelling can lead to mom feeling very uncomfortable and can even make moving hurt. Edema is best addressed through topical use of essential oils, such as a massage oil or an epsom salt bath. Massaging an essential oil blend in can be very calming and relaxing. By using a therapeutic blend that increases circulation or helps with edema, you can multiply the benefits. Essential oils that may help include cypress, grapefruit, juniper berry, rosemary, mandarin, orange, and tangerine.

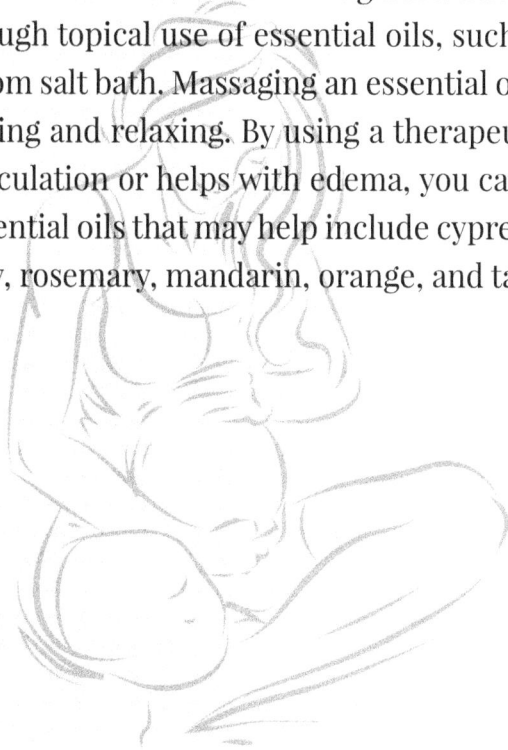

## Edema Massage Oil

**What You Will Need:**

> 5 drops cypress essential oil
>
> 5 drops grapefruit essential oil
>
> 2 drops rosemary essential oil
>
> 2 tablespoons olive oil
>
> 2-ounce amber glass dropper bottle

**What To Do:**

1. Add essential oils and a carrier oil to the bottle.

2. Replace dropper top and shake to mix well.

**To Use:** Place five to ten drops into your palm and use deep massaging motions to move oil toward the heart for five minutes. Elevate your legs by propping them up with a cushion.

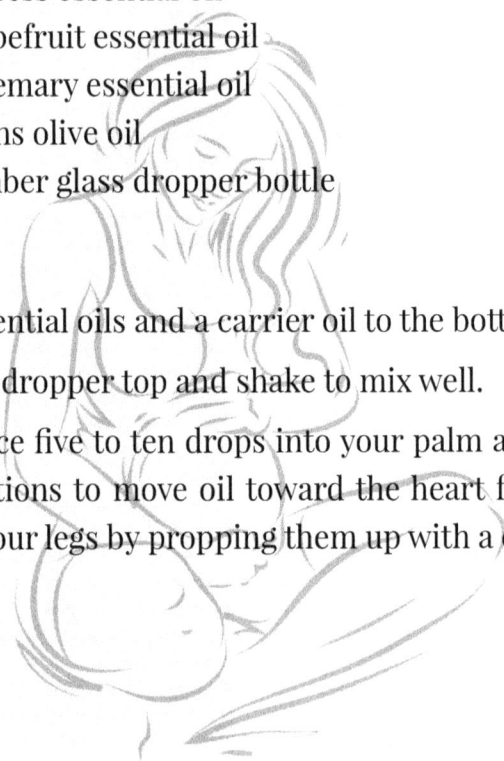

## *Edema Foot Soak*

**What You Will Need:**

¼ cup epsom salts
10 drops grapefruit essential oil
10 drops cypress essential oil
foot bathtub

**What To Do:**

1. In a glass cup, add epsom salts and essential oils. Stir to mix well.

2. Fill a foot bath with hot water. Add salts and swirl around to dissolve in the water.

**To Use:** Soak feet for 15 minutes to help reduce swelling. Repeat every week or two to alleviate pain from swollen ankles and feet. Elevate feet on a stool afterward.

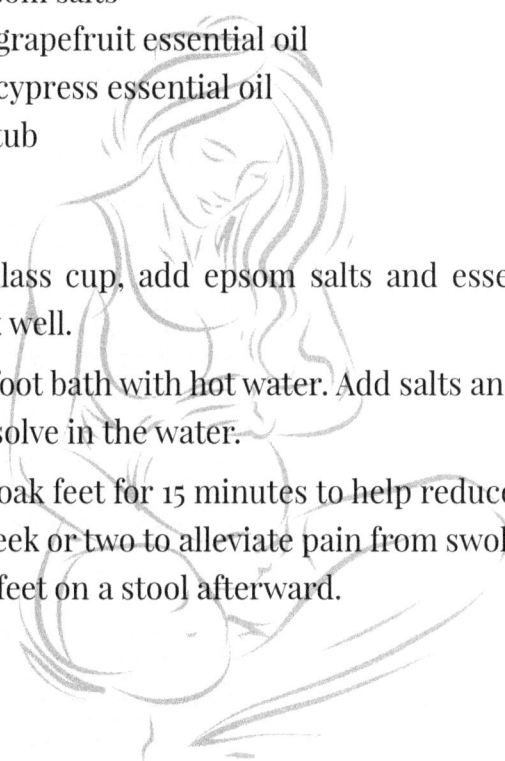

## Edema Ankle Rub

**What You Will Need:**

> 10 drops juniper berry essential oil
> 10 drops mandarin essential oil
> 10 drops geranium essential oil
> 10 drops cypress essential oil
> 4 tablespoons coconut oil
> 4-ounce amber glass dropper bottle

**What To Do:**

1. In a glass bottle, add all essential oils and carrier oil.

2. Replace top and shake to blend.

**To Use:** Place a dime-size amount in your palm and massage into your ankles and feet. Use weekly—this is concentrated.

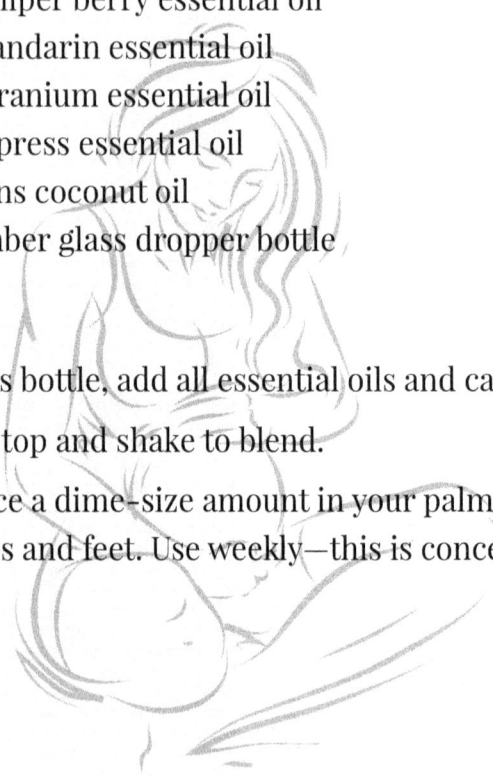

# Fetal Positioning

During pregnancy, the developing baby moves into several different positions. As labor approaches, some positions are safer than others. The ideal position for a fetus just before labor is the anterior position. In this position, the fetus's head points toward the ground and they are facing the woman's back — most fetuses settle into this position by the last month of pregnancy. The anterior position is also known as a vertex, cephalic, or occiput anterior position. The anterior position may reduce the chances of complications during pregnancy.

Baby doesn't always want to be positioned the way that we may want him or her to be when it comes time to prepare for birth. Applying diluted essential oils topically to the top part of the uterus may be useful in helping the baby to position itself correctly. Essential oils that may help include peppermint, pine, spearmint, and siberian fir.

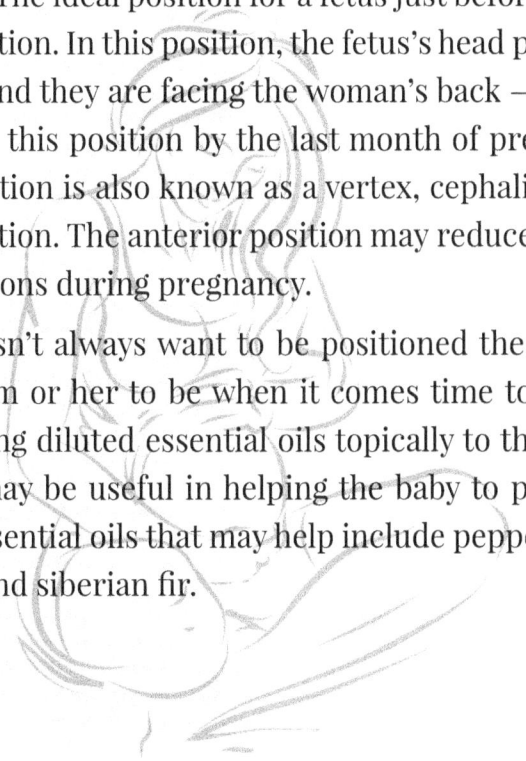

## Moving Baby Blend

**What You Will Need:**

5 drops myrrh essential oil

5 drops peppermint essential oil

1 tablespoon fractionated coconut oil

**What To Do:**

1. Pour a tablespoon of coconut oil into your palm.

2. Add the essential oils and mix with finger.

**To Use:** Rub into the belly. Repeat as needed to help the baby turn around.

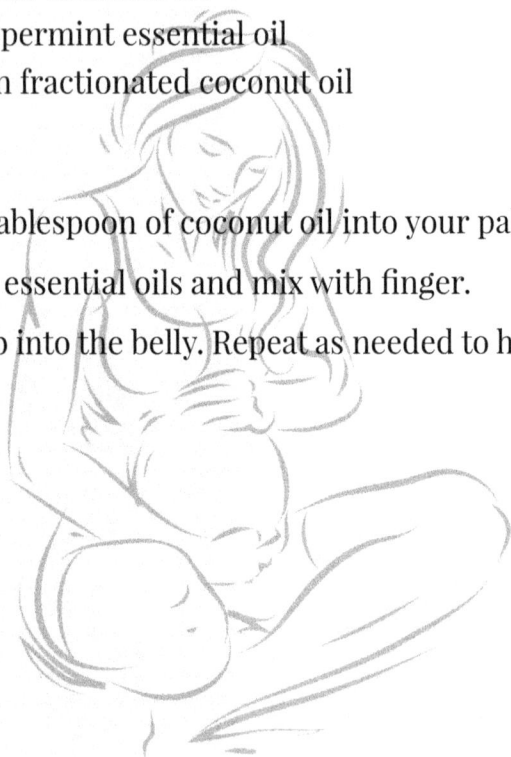

# Group B Strep/Bacterial Vaginosis

Sometimes, bacterial infections can occur during pregnancy. It's important to treat these promptly. Making a vaginal pessary or an aromatic bath would be the ideal choice for essential oil use here. Essential oils that may help include lavender and tea tree.

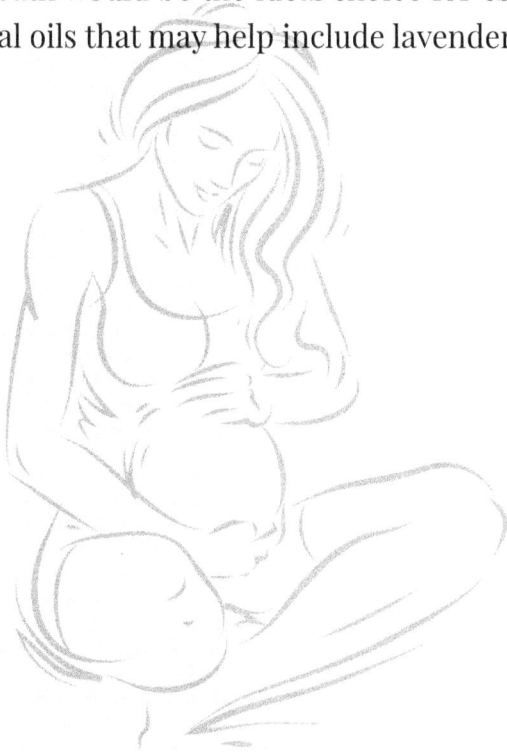

## Group B Strep Blend

**What You Will Need:**

9 drops lavender essential oil
15 drops tea tree essential oil
1 teaspoon coconut oil
cotton tampon

**What To Do:**

1. In a glass bowl, mix the essential oils with the coconut oil.

2. Soak a tampon in the mixture overnight.

**To Use:** Wear overnight and wash area in shower in the morning. Do this daily for the last six weeks of pregnancy.

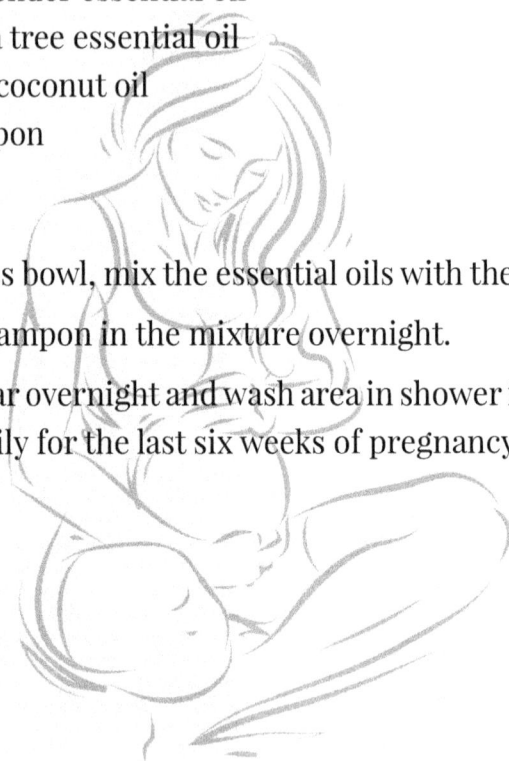

## *Bacterial Vaginosis Salve*

**What You Will Need:**

¼ cup coconut oil
¼ cup cocoa butter
2 tablespoons calendula oil
½ teaspoon thyme or oregano essential oil
2 tablespoons goldenseal powder
1 tablespoon myrrh powder
small saucepan
silicone suppository mold

**What To Do:**

1. In a small saucepan, melt ¼ cup of coconut oil and ¼ cup of cocoa butter.

2. Remove from heat and add calendula oil, essential oil, goldenseal powder, and myrrh powder.

3. Pour the warm, slightly thick liquid into a suppository mold.

4. Place the mold into the fridge and let the suppositories harden for about an hour.

5. Pop the suppositories out, place in a clean jar, and store in the refrigerator until ready to use.

**To Use:** Insert into the vagina before bed once a night. Be sure to get retested to check the progress of treatment.

# Headache

Headaches can occur for a variety of reasons in pregnancy, including hormonal changes, vascular dilation, or even dehydration. To treat headaches with essential oils, either a roller bottle remedy or inhalation would be the best routes of delivery. Essential oils that may help include eucalyptus, Roman chamomile, lavender, lemon, neroli, and peppermint.

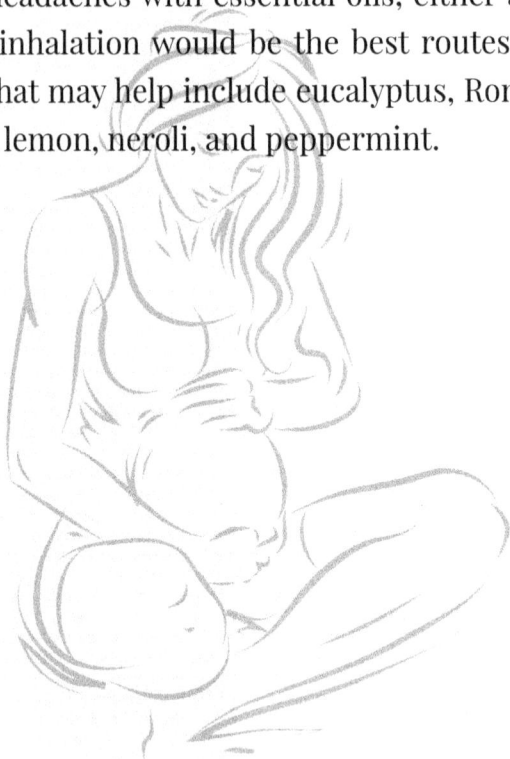

## Headache Salve

**What You Will Need:**

> 2/3 cup almond or jojoba oil
> 1/3 cup beeswax
> 1/4 cup coconut oil
> 4 drops vitamin E oil
> 8 drops peppermint essential oil
> 3 drops eucalyptus essential oil (optional)
> 2 4-ounce mason jars

**What To Do:**

1. In a double boiler, add almond oil, beeswax, and coconut oil. Heat until completely melted.

2. Take the mixture off of the heat and allow cooling for a minute or two.

3. Stir in the vitamin E oil and essential oils.

4. Pour mixture into small mason jars and allow to cool before replacing the top.

# Heartburn

The slowing of digestion or pressure on the stomach from a growing uterus can both lead to heartburn. The burning pain in your chest behind your breastbone is often worse after eating, in the evening, or when lying down or bending over. Occasional heartburn is common and no cause for alarm. Most moms-to-be can manage the discomfort of heartburn on their own with essential oils. It is recommended to apply a massage oil over the neck, chest, and upper abdomen for help in treating heartburn with essential oils. Essential oils that may help include black pepper, cajeput, German chamomile, Roman chamomile, cypress, eucalyptus, ginger, mandarin, neroli, peppermint, and spearmint.

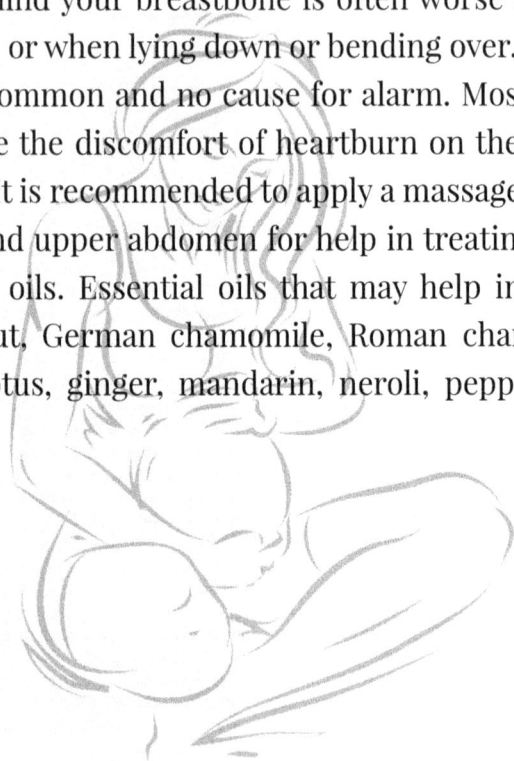

## *Heartburn Relief Roll-On*

**What You Will Need:**

10 drops neroli essential oil
10 drops petitgrain essential oil
15 drops orange essential oil
5 drops lavender essential oil
10 ml roller bottle

**What To Do:**

1. Remove the ball and add essential oils to it. Replace ball and cap.

2. Shake to blend.

**To Use:** Roll the oil over neck and chest as needed.

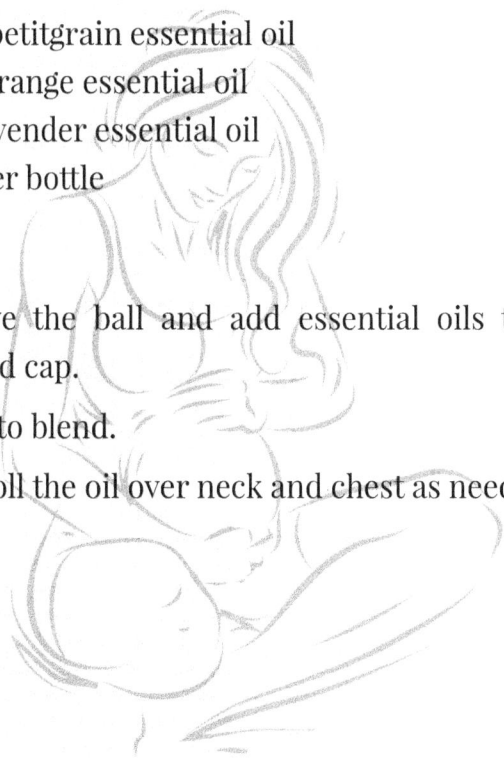

## Heartburn Quick Relief Oil

**What You Will Need:**

10 drops coriander essential oil
5 drops grapefruit essential oil
4 drops ginger essential oil
5 drops lemon essential oil
2 ounces fractionated coconut oil
2-ounce amber glass dropper bottle

**What To Do:**

1.  Add the essential oils into the glass dropper bottle.

2.  Replace cap and shake gently to blend.

**To Use:** Place five to seven drops of the heartburn blend onto your palm, rub your palms together, and apply it to your abdomen and chest in gentle circular motions.

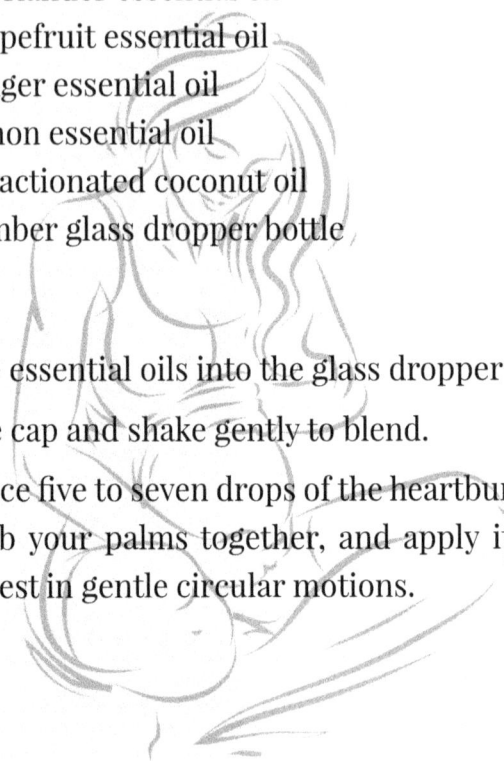

# Hemorrhoids

Due to constipation, or even pushing during delivery, hemorrhoids can occur. Hemorrhoids, also called piles, are swollen veins in your anus and lower rectum, similar to varicose veins. Hemorrhoids have a number of causes, although often the cause is unknown. They may result from straining during bowel movements or from the increased pressure on these veins during pregnancy. Hemorrhoids may be located inside the rectum (internal hemorrhoids), or they may develop under the skin around the anus (external hemorrhoids). Hemorrhoids are very common. Sometimes they don't cause symptoms but at other times they cause itching, discomfort, and bleeding. A rectal suppository, spray, or salve are all excellent usage choices. It is recommended to use moist wipes instead of toilet paper for cleansing. A warm sitz bath can also alleviate the discomfort from swollen veins. Soak for 20-30 minutes if possible. Essential oils that may help include cypress, frankincense, lavender, juniper berry, geranium, helichrysum, orange, and sandalwood.

## Postpartum Healing Padsicles

**What You Will Need:**

10 overnight maxi pads
½ cup witch hazel
½ cup aloe vera gel
10 drops lavender essential oil
1 ounce comfrey leaves
2 cups boiling water

**What To Do:**

1. Boil water and pour over comfrey tea leaves. Cover and steep for 8 hours.

2. Strain comfrey leaves and set aside the tea.

3. In a medium bowl, add tea, witch hazel, aloe vera gel, and lavender essential oil.

4. Open each maxi pad, leaving in its wrapper.

5. Pour 2-4 tablespoons of the mixture over each pad, concentrating on where your sore perineum will be.

6. Refold pad and close up. Wrap in foil and place in a gallon-size freezer bag. Place in the freezer until ready for use.

**To Use:** Remove pad from the freezer and let thaw for five minutes before use. Wear as needed for soothing comfort.

## Homemade Tucks Pads

**What You Will Need:**

1 cup witch hazel (alcohol-free)
½ cup aloe vera juice
2-4 teaspoons helichrysum hydrosol (or substitute: German chamomile hydrosol)
1 package cotton rounds
large glass jar

**What To Do:**

1. In a glass jar, place as many cotton rounds as you can fit. Set aside.

2. In a glass measuring cup, add all of the liquid ingredients. Stir well. Pour over the cotton rounds slowly until all pads are soaked.

3. Seal and store in the refrigerator, or the bathroom for the few days needed.

## Peri Wipe Spray

**What You Will Need:**

5 drops geranium essential oil

4 drops lavender essential oil

3 drops orange essential oil

40 drops fractionated coconut oil

pre-moistened wipes or unscented diaper wipes

**What To Do:**

1. In a glass spray bottle, add essential oils and coconut oil.

2. Replace sprayer top and shake to blend.

**To Use:** When ready to use, squirt two or three sprays on a pre-moistened wipe. Use instead of toilet paper.

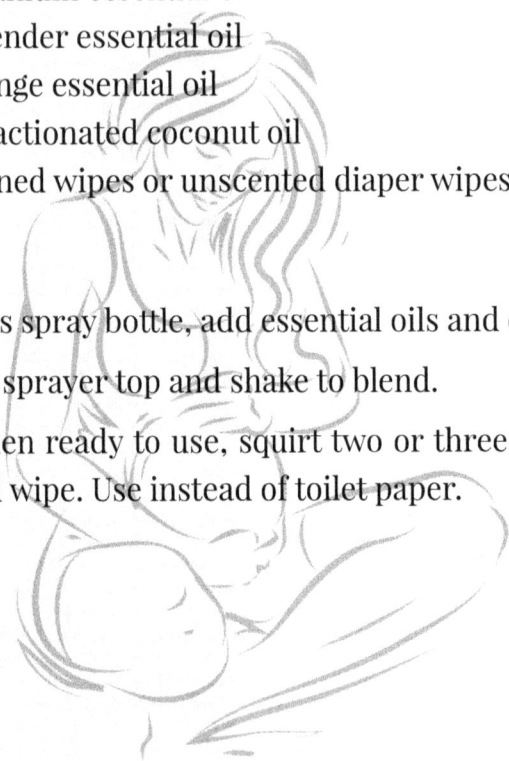

## *Peri Spray*

**What You Will Need:**

> 1 teaspoon witch hazel (alcohol-free)
> 2 drops cypress essential oil
> 2 drops juniper berry essential oil
> 2 drops geranium essential oil
> 8 teaspoons aloe vera juice (unscented)

**What To Do:**

1. In a glass spray bottle, combine witch hazel and essential oils and mix well.

2. Next, add unscented aloe vera gel. Shake to blend.

3. Store in refrigerator until ready for use.

**To Use:** Spray on a wipe to cleanse the area. Or, spray on a pad to wear.

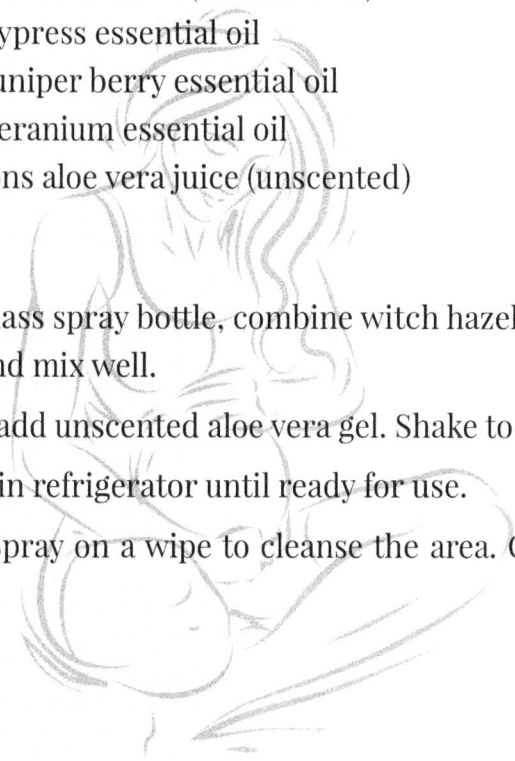

# Insomnia

Sleeping can be difficult for a pregnant woman. Besides having to use the bathroom more frequently, the growing uterus makes it difficult to get comfortable. Wrestling with not being able to sleep in a normal position may also lead to sleeplessness. Aromatic use is the best mode of delivery when dealing with insomnia. Essential oils that may help include bergamot, Roman chamomile, lavender, lemon, neroli, petitgrain, orange, sandalwood, and vetiver.

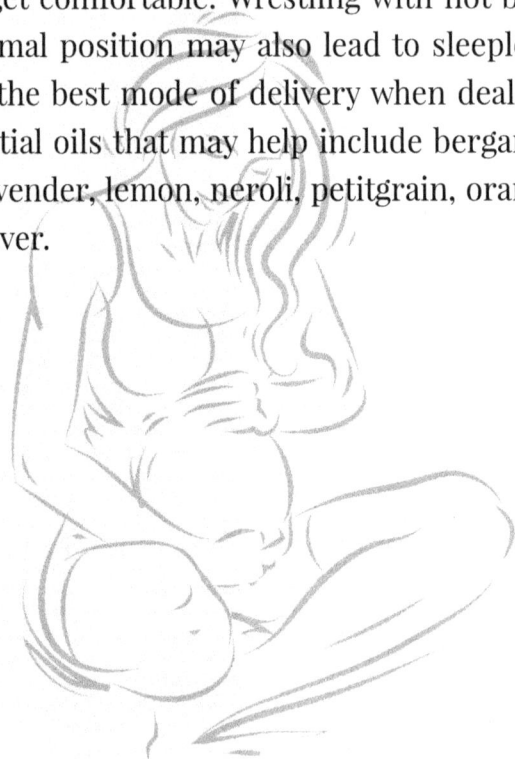

## *Sleepy Time Diffuser Blend*

**What You Will Need:**

10 drops lavender essential oil
10 drops frankincense essential oil
10 drops cedarwood essential oil
10 drops bergamot essential oil
5 ml dark-colored bottle with lid
diffuser

**What To Do:**

1. Combine all oils into a small, dark-colored bottle.

2. Close the cap the bottle tightly and shake well to blend.

3. Follow directions for your diffuser and add water as needed.

4. Add about ten drops of your blend into your diffuser.

**To Use:** Place in your bedroom at night and run for a few minutes before bedtime. Other combinations include:

| | |
|---|---|
| Dreamcatcher | Clary Sage and Cedarwood |
| Dreamland | Cedarwood, Lavender, and Ravensara |
| Sleeping Beauty | Bergamot, Lavender, and Marjoram |
| Mr. Sandman | Clary Sage, Lavender, and Vetiver |
| Naptime | Marjoram, Neroli, and Patchouli |
| Chill Pill | Orange, Roman Chamomile, and Lavender |
| Winter Slumber | Frankincense, Orange, and Patchouli |
| Five More Minutes | Orange, Lavender, and Marjoram |

## *Sweet Dreams Roll-On*

**What You Will Need:**

>   1 drop neroli essential oil
>   1 drop vetiver essential oil
>   3 drops cedarwood essential oil
>   3 drops sandalwood essential oil
>   fractionated coconut oil
>   10 ml roll-on bottle

**What To Do:**

1.  Remove the ball from the roller bottle and add essential oils and carrier oil.

2.  Replace cap and shake to blend.

**To Use:** Roll this blend onto your feet, your neck/forehead/shoulders before retiring to bed. Or, you can use essential oils only in a diffuser blend fifteen minutes before sleep.

# Leg Cramp

Leg cramps during pregnancy can be downright unbearable and lead to loss of mobility and sleeplessness. It can be common and usually harmless condition where the muscles in your leg suddenly become tight and painful. Leg cramps typically occur in the calf muscles, although it can affect any part of your leg, including your feet and thighs. After the cramping has passed, you may have pain and tenderness in your leg for several hours.

Making a massage oil or lotion that can be rubbed into the cramping muscles is very effective for leg cramps. Essential oils that may help include Roman chamomile, copaiba, cypress (after 20 weeks gestation), geranium, lavender, and peppermint.

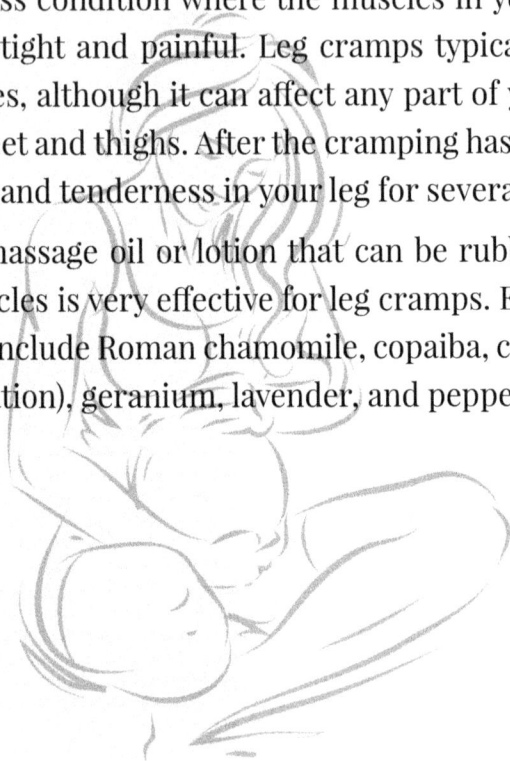

101315192123273335373941454749515355576265687073757881858891101104106111113116118121123131133137139141143146148150152154156158160161

## *Leg Cramp Massage Oil*

**What You Will Need:**

- 1 teaspoon olive oil
- 1 teaspoon coconut oil
- 1 drop bergamot essential oil
- 2 drops rosemary ct. camphor essential oil
- 15 ml dark glass bottle

**What To Do:**

1. Add all of the oils together in the glass bottle.

2. Shake to mix well.

**To Use**: Apply on the cramping area and massage for five minutes to relieve the tension and pain.

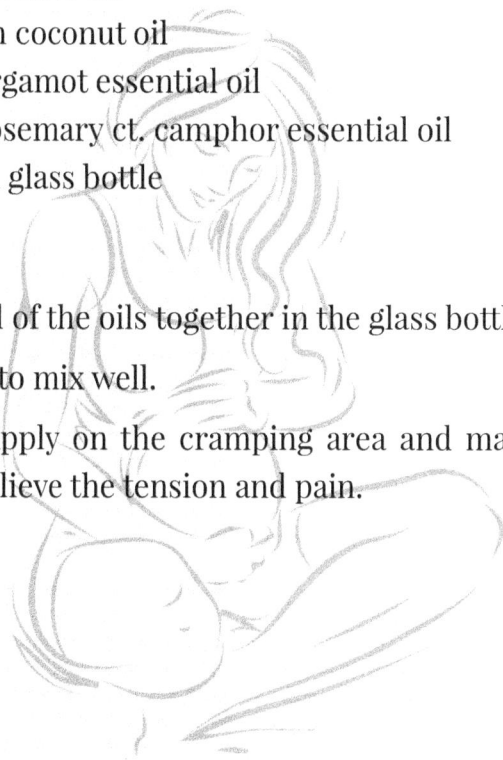

## Leg Cramp Relief

**What You Will Need:**

> 1 tablespoon olive oil
> ½ tablespoon tamanu oil
> 5 drops wintergreen essential oil
> 10 drops cypress essential oil

**What To Do:**

1. In a glass bottle, add all oils together.

2. Shake to mix well before each use.

**To Use:** Apply the blend on the legs morning and evening, covering the most prone area. This blend can also be used to prevent leg cramps. Simply massage on your legs for a few minutes each day as needed.

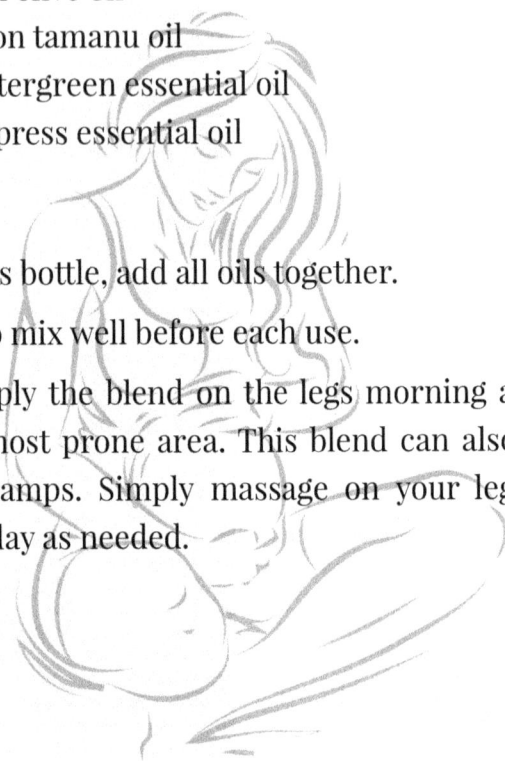

# Charley Horse

Charley horse is another name for a muscle spasm. Charley horses can occur in any muscle, but they're most common in the legs. These spasms are marked by uncomfortable muscle contractions. If the contracting muscles don't relax for several seconds or more, the pain can be severe. Severe charley horses can result in muscle soreness that lasts anywhere from a few hours to a day. This is normal, so long as the pain isn't prolonged or recurring. Charley horses are generally treatable at home, especially if they're infrequent. However, frequent muscle spasms are often linked to underlying health conditions that need medical treatment.

Making a massage oil or lotion that can be rubbed into the cramping muscles is very effective for charley horses. Essential oils that may help include Roman chamomile, copaiba, cypress (after 20 weeks gestation), eucalyptus, geranium, lavender, rosemary, and peppermint.

## Charley Horse Salve

**What You Will Need:**

¼ cup olive oil
¼ cup shea butter
1 tablespoon beeswax pellets
20 drops rosemary essential oil
15 drops peppermint essential oil
10 drops eucalyptus essential oil
10 drops cypress essential oil
small mason jar with lid

**What To Do:**

1. Melt the olive oil, shea butter, and beeswax pellets in a glass jar in the microwave or a double boiler.

2. Remove from heat when completely melted, then let sit for a few minutes to cool. Add the essential oils and stir to combine.

3. Pour the mixture into a lidded jar and let harden in the refrigerator for 20 minutes. Store in a cool, dry place up to one year.

**To Use:** Massage a small amount of muscle rub onto the affected area for relief.

## *Charley Horse Salve #2*

**What You Will Need:**

¼ cup almond oil

¼ cup coconut oil

1 tablespoon beeswax pellets

7 drops clove essential oil

7 drops peppermint essential oil

7 drops lavender essential oil

7 drops eucalyptus essential oil

7 drops rosemary essential oil

7 drops copaiba essential oil

small mason jar with lid

**What To Do:**

1. In a double boiler, combine the almond oil, coconut oil, and beeswax pellets. Heat at medium until melted. Whisk to completely mix.

2. Remove from heat and let cool on the counter for about three minutes. Add the essential oils to the mixture and whisk to blend well.

**To Use:** Apply on the affected area as needed.

# Nausea and Vomiting

The hormonal changes going on in a pregnant woman's body can lead to nausea and vomiting, sometimes touted as morning sickness. However, we know that it can happen at any time of the day or last all day. Aromatic use is great if the mom can handle the smell of the oils. Otherwise, a massage oil for over the stomach can help. Essential oils that can help include black pepper, cardamom, German chamomile, Roman chamomile, ginger, and peppermint.

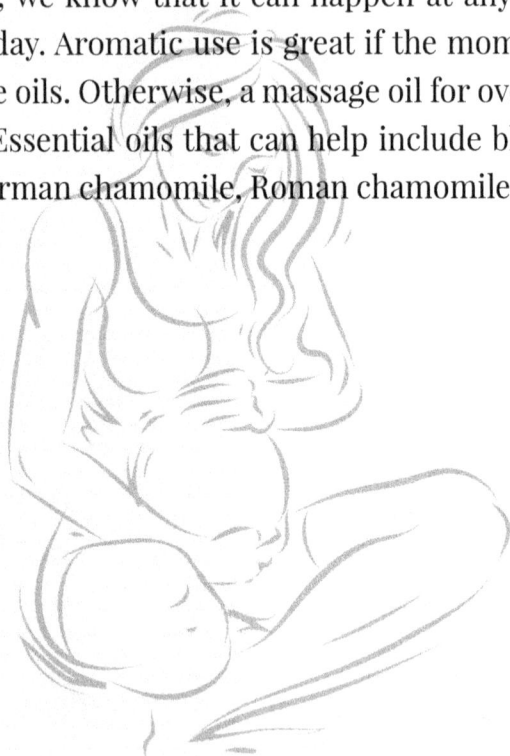

## *Nausea Inhaler*

Morning sickness or nausea (with or without vomiting) can strike at any time of the day or night. It often begins one month after you become pregnant. However, some women feel nausea earlier and others never experience it. While the cause of nausea during pregnancy isn't clear, pregnancy hormones likely play a role.

**What You Will Need:**

inhaler

5 drops ginger essential oil

5 drops lemon essential oil

5 drops mandarin essential oil

glass bowl

tweezers

**What To Do:**

1. Place five drops each of ginger, lemon, and mandarin into a glass bowl.

2. Place the wick from the inhaler into the bowl with the essential oils and use the tweezers to move the wick around to absorb the essential oils.

3. Once the wick has absorbed all of the oil, use the tweezers to pick up the wick and place it inside the inhaler tube.

4. Snap the bottom on and replace the cap on the inhaler.

5. Label the inhaler.

**To Use:** Waft under the nose and take a deep breath during times of nausea.

## Nausea Salts

**What You Will Need:**

1 tablespoon sea salts
6 drops ginger essential oil
1 drop peppermint essential oil
dark-colored glass bottle

**What To Do:**

1. In a dark-colored glass bottle, add the sea salts along with the essential oils.

2. Shake to blend well.

**To Use:** Inhale from the bottle when feeling nauseous or have a stomach upset.

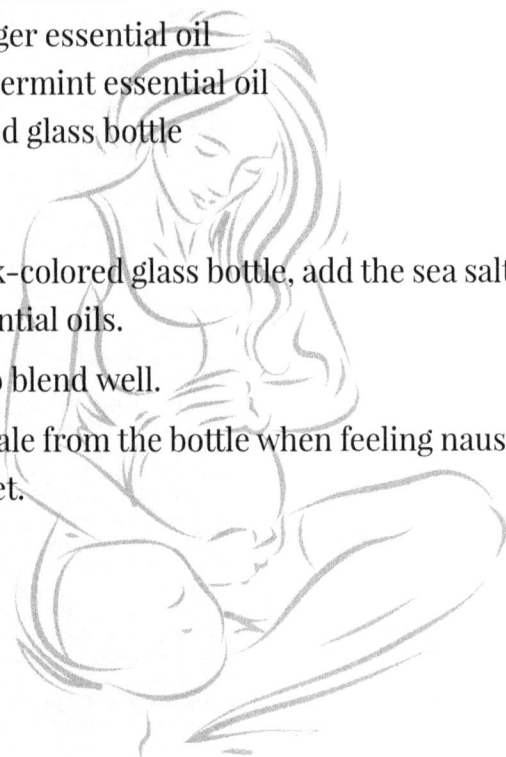

## *Nausea Diffuser Blend*

**What Will You Need:**

> 2 drops peppermint essential oil
> 2 drops bergamot essential oil
> 2 drops chamomile essential oil

**What To Do:**

1. Add your peppermint, bergamot, and chamomile to your diffuser water. Add more as needed.

2. Turn the diffuser on, and let it run for 15 minutes of every hour.

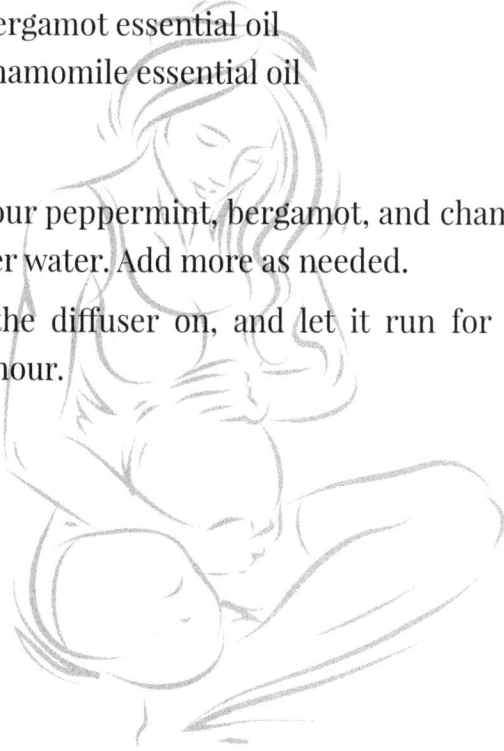

## Soothing Tummy Bath Blend

**What You Will Need:**

> 3 drops bergamot essential oil
> 3 drops chamomile essential oil
> ½ cup sea salts

**What To Do:**

1. In a small bowl, blend essential oils and salts together.

2. Pour under running water and swish around to blend.

**To Use:** Soak in the bathwater until the water cools to body temp. Inhale deeply — Repeat as necessary until your nausea has subsided.

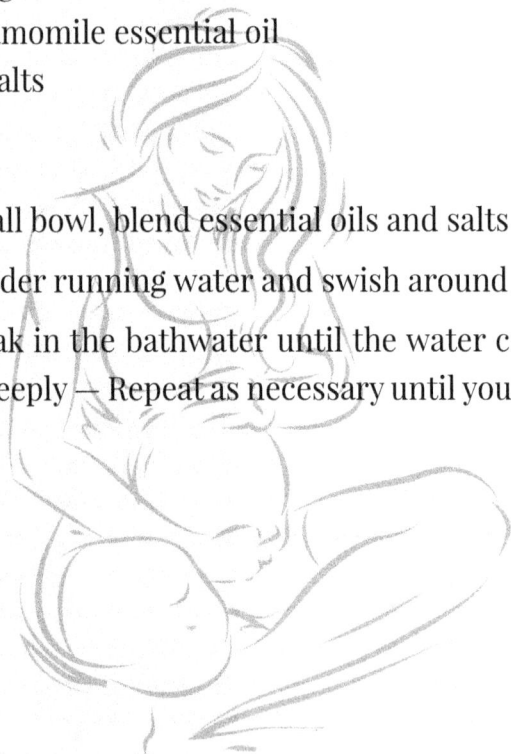

# Preeclampsia

This can make a mom's blood pressure rise to dangerous levels. Aromatic support should be handled aromatically and focus on helping the mom to destress and relax. Essential oils that may help include bergamot, Roman chamomile, frankincense, geranium, lavender, lemon, lime, orange, and sandalwood.

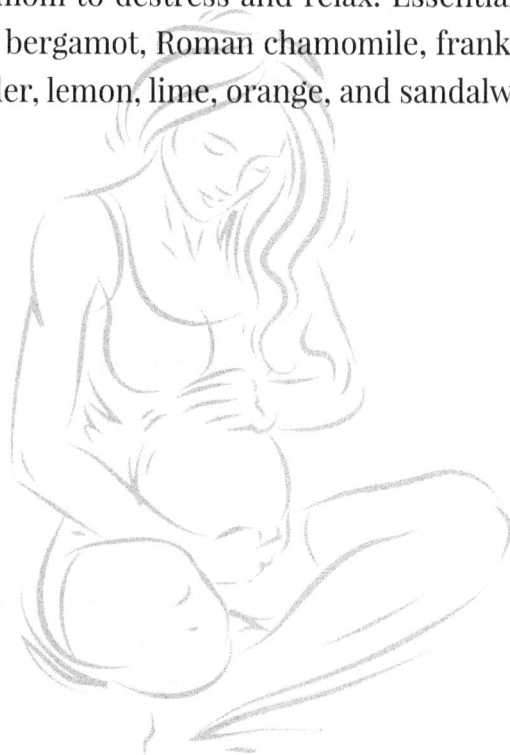

## *Lemon Oil Water*

**What You Will Need:**

lemon essential oil

**What To Do:**

1.  Put two or three drops of the essential oil of lemon in a bottle or a glass of water.

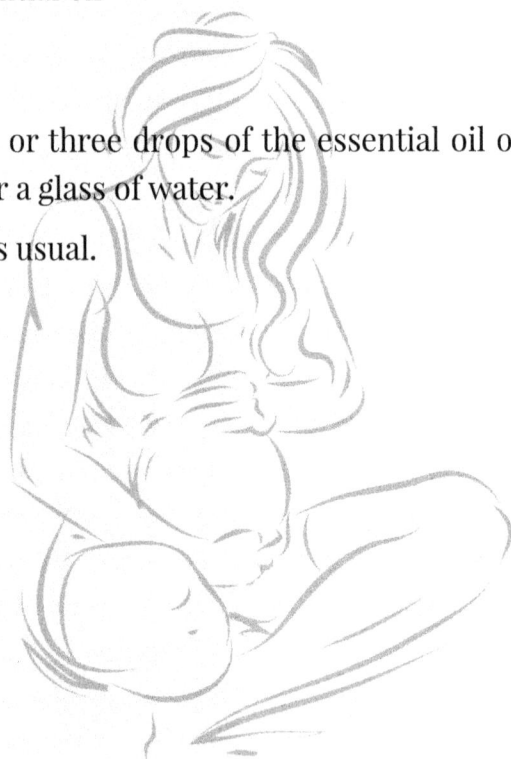

2.  Drink as usual.

## *Preeclampsia Bath Blend*

**What You Will Need:**

> 1 drop sandalwood essential oil
> 2 drops geranium essential oil
> 2 drops lavender essential oil
> ½ cup sea salts

**What To Do:**

1. In a small container, add salts and essential oils. Stir to blend.

2. Add to running bath water.

**To Use:** Soak in the bath for at least 20 minutes. This mixture soothes and calms the nerves to relieve stress and body pressure.

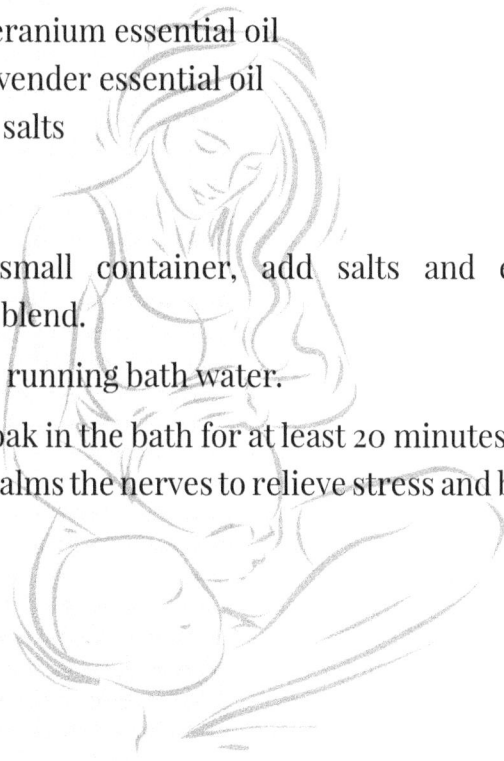

# Fatigue

It's common to feel extremely tired during the first 12 weeks of your pregnancy. With hormonal changes, the emotional roller-coaster and extra weight can leave you exhausted. Fatigue is an overall feeling of tiredness or lack of energy. It isn't the same as simply feeling drowsy or sleepy. When you're fatigued, you have no motivation and no energy. Being sleepy may be a symptom of fatigue, but it's not the same thing. Fatigue is a common symptom of many medical conditions that range in severity from mild to serious. It's also a natural result of some lifestyle choices, such as lack of exercise or poor diet. Using essential oils aromatically can help the mom-to-be get a little more energy back. Essential oils that may help include geranium, grapefruit, lavender, lemon, peppermint, and orange.

After the birth of the baby, you may experience fatigue from being up at all hours of the night, trying to recover from giving birth, and having a new little life dependent on you can make mom one tired person. Support her aromatically by using essential oils in a personal inhaler that she can use as needed. In addition to the essential oils listed above, you will want to include bergamot, lime, rosemary, and spearmint.

## *Fatigue Salve*

**What You Will Need:**

½ cup coconut oil
¼ cup beeswax pellets (or grated)
2 teaspoons cayenne powder
2 teaspoons ginger powder
15 drops peppermint essential oil
15 drops lavender essential oil
glass jar

**What To Do:**

1. Add coconut oil and beeswax to a jar. Place a saucepan with two inches of water over medium-low heat.

2. Allow contents to melt. Stir to combine. Add the cayenne and ginger powder and stir well.

3. Allow mixture to cool slightly, then add in essential oils — mix well.

4. Pour mixture into metal tins or storage containers and allow to set.

## *Fatigue Massage Oil*

**What You Will Need:**

10 ml evening primrose oil
2 drops clary sage essential oil
2 drops frankincense essential oil
2 drops lavender essential oil
2 drops neroli essential oil
1 drops ylang ylang essential oil
10 ml roller bottle

**What To Do:**

1. In a roller bottle, add the essential oils then fill the remaining space with a carrier oil.

2. Replace ball and cap and shake well.

**To Use:** Massage over neck (thyroid) and along lower back/over kidneys (adrenals) morning and night.

# Flatulence

Being pregnant can come along with a lot of gas and discomfort associated with gas. Flatulence can be managed through either aromatic or topical use of essential oils. Essential oils that may help with this include black pepper, cardamom, cumin, dill seed, ginger, lavender, peppermint, roman chamomile, and spearmint.

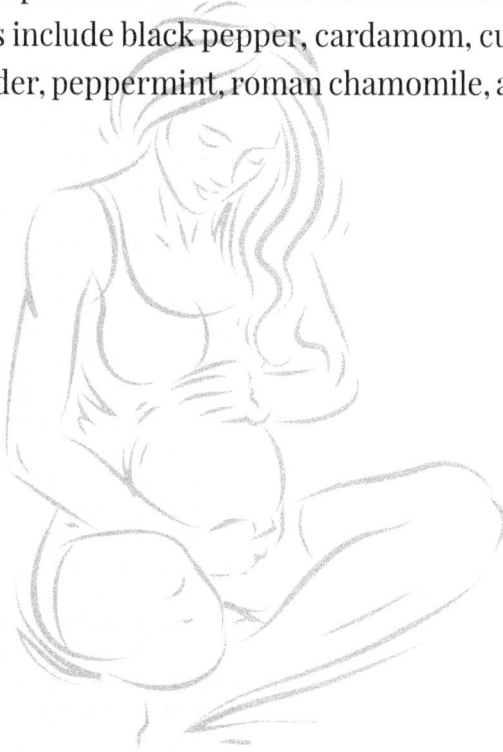

## *Deflate Roll-on*

**What You Will Need:**

2 drops peppermint essential oil
2 drops cumin essential oil
2 drops ginger essential oil
½ ounce jojoba oil
10 ml roller bottle

**What To Do:**

1. In a roller bottle, add essential oils then fill the remaining space with a carrier oil.

2. Replace ball and cap and shake well.

**To Use:** Roll over lower abdomen and intestines as needed.

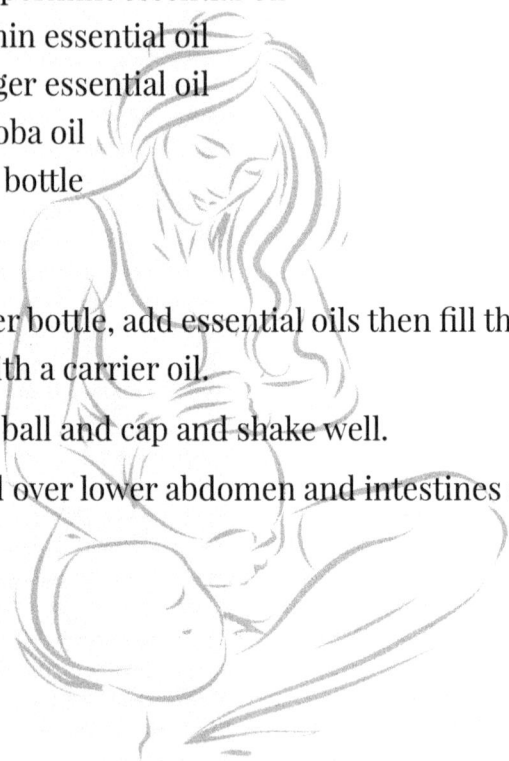

## Gas-X Massage Oil

**What You Will Need:**

    5 drops cardamom essential oil
    4 drops grapefruit essential oil
    2 drops black pepper essential oil
    ½ ounce almond oil
    15 ml glass bottle

**What To Do:**

In a glass bottle, add essential oils. Fill the remaining space with the carrier oil.

Replace cap and shake well.

**To Use:** Place several drops into your palm and massage into your lower abdomen and over the intestines in a circular motion. Use as needed.

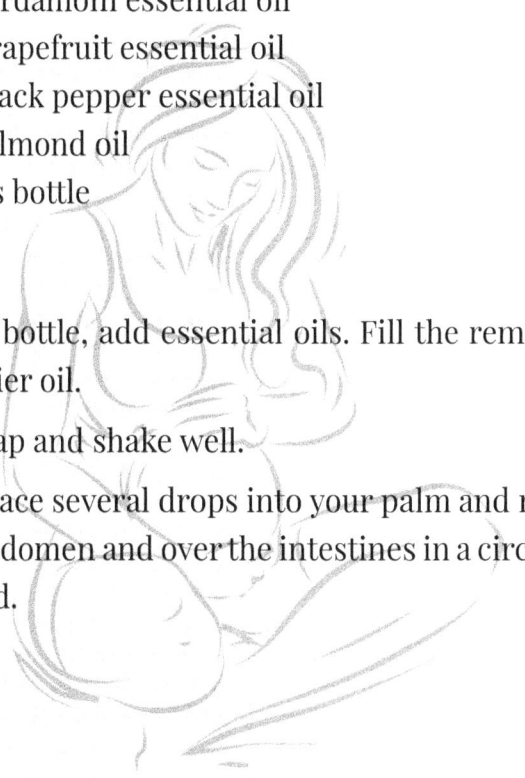

# PUPPS (pruritic urticarial papules and plaques of pregnancy)

A rash can sometimes develop during pregnancy due to rapid weight gain. The skin is rapidly stretched, which can lead to inflammation. If you are dealing with PUPPS, you'll want to use a topical approach with your essential oils. Essential oils that may help include German chamomile, Roman chamomile, lavender, helichrysum, patchouli, and sandalwood.

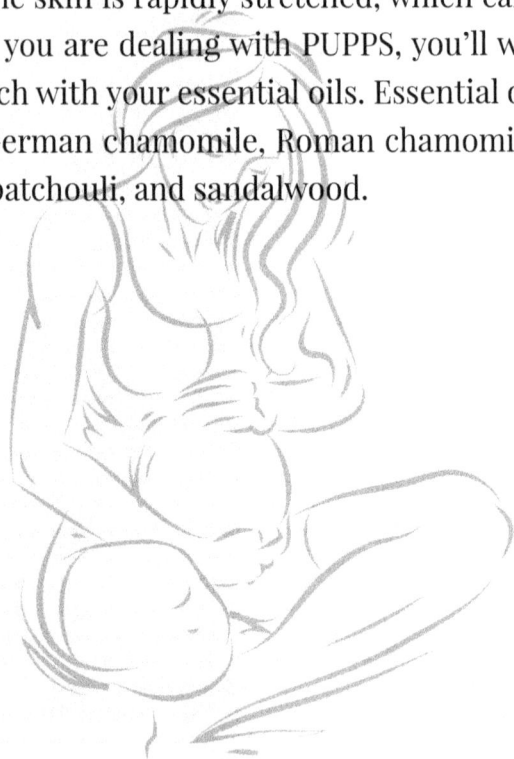

## PUPPS Roll-On

**What You Will Need:**

10 drops peppermint essential oil
5 drops lavender essential oil
5 drops geranium essential oil
4 drops frankincense essential oil
4 drops German chamomile essential oil
2 drops ylang ylang essential oil
2 drops eucalyptus essential oil
2 drops tea tree essential oil
1 ounce organic jojoba oil
glass roller bottle

**What To Do:**

1. In a glass bottle, add essential oils and jojoba oil until full.

2. Replace the cap with roller top and shake to blend.

**To Use:** For immediate relief, apply as needed. Test this blend on a small patch of skin first and avoid use in sensitive areas such as the groin, armpits, nipples, and mucous membranes.

# Round Ligament Pain

As the uterus grows, the ligaments surround the uterus have to stretch to accommodate this growth, which results in round ligament pain. Round ligament pain is best addressed by topical use of essential oils. Essential oils that may help include black pepper, Roman chamomile, and lavender.

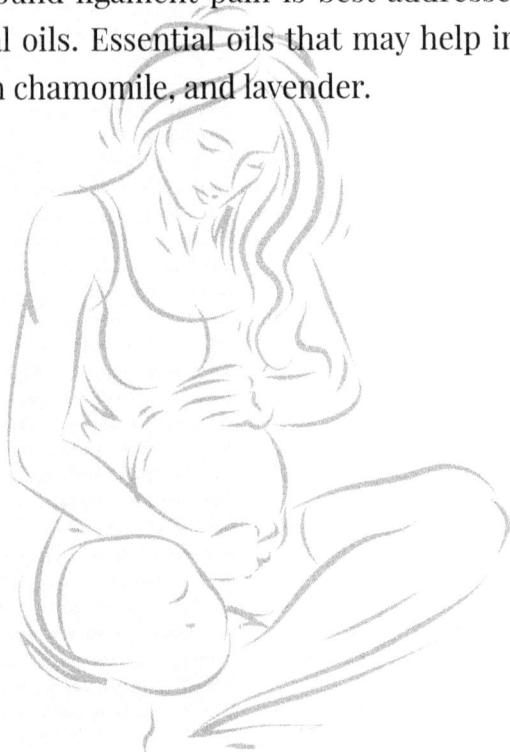

## *Tummy Rub*

**What You Will Need:**

2 drops Roman chamomile essential oil
2 drops lavender essential oil
1 teaspoon fractionated coconut oil
5 ml glass bottle

**What To Do:**

1.  In a glass bottle, add essential oils and coconut oil.

2.  Replace cap and shake to blend.

**To Use:** Rub over the tummy as needed.

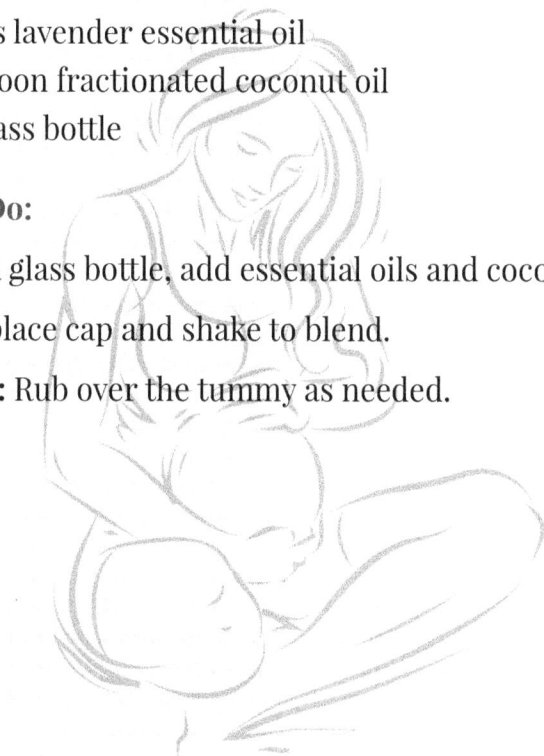

# Sciatica

The sciatic nerve can become compressed during pregnancy, leading to a great deal of discomfort for mom. Sciatica refers to pain that radiates along the path of the sciatic nerve, which branches from your lower back through your hips and buttocks and down each leg. Typically, sciatica affects only one side of your body. Sciatica can best be addressed through topical use of essential oils. Essential oils that may help include black pepper, cajeput, German chamomile, eucalyptus, ginger, lavender, nutmeg, and peppermint.

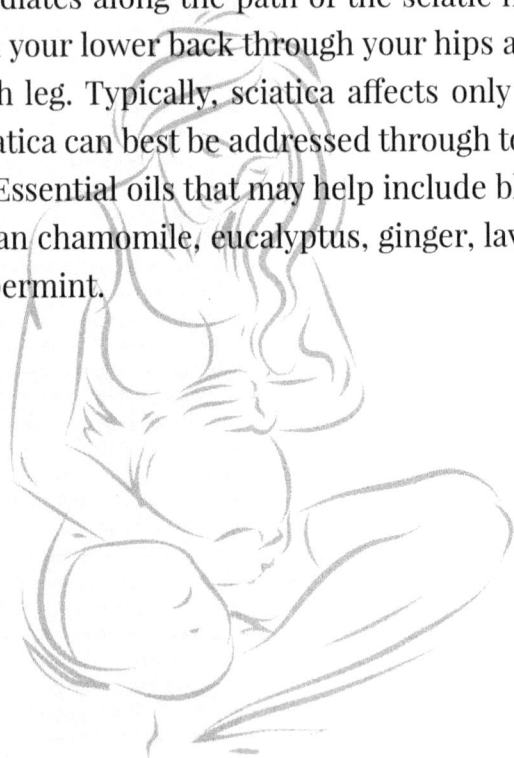

## *Sciatica Cool Compress*

**What You Will Need:**

10 drops lavender essential oil
10 drops ginger essential oil
5 drops marjoram essential oil
5 drops rosemary essential oil
1 teaspoon almond oil
5 ml glass bottle

**What To Do:**

1. In a 5 ml glass dropper bottle, combine your essential oils, and almond oil.

2. Shake to blend.

3. When using as a cold compress, use a small bowl, and combine two cups of cold water with 12 drops of your blend. Stir well.

4. Soak a cloth in the mixture. Wring out your towel and place on painful areas of your lower back. Apply once every two hours, alternating a cold pack between cloth application.

**To Use:** You can also use as a massage oil by gently rubbing over the back. For the bath, fill the tub with warm water and add 10-12 drops of the blend. Agitate the water to disperse the oil. Soak in the tub for at least 20 minutes or more.

## *Sciatica Salve*

**What You Will Need:**

1 cup olive oil
¾ ounce rosemary (dried or fresh)
¼ ounce cayenne pepper
½ ounce beeswax
¼ teaspoon vitamin E oil
4 drops peppermint essential oil
1 drop wintergreen essential oil
glass measuring cup
cheesecloth or coffee filter
Salve tins or jars

**What To Do:**

1. Grind the rosemary and cayenne pepper into a fine powder. In a separate container with lid, add one cup of olive oil.

2. Add dry herbs in the olive oil. Let sit for one to four weeks. Give a good shake once a day.

3. When ready, fill a pot halfway with water and place glass measuring cup inside the pan. Heat water at medium heat.

4. Strain olive oil mixture through a cheesecloth or coffee filter into a clean bowl.

5. Add infused olive oil to the measuring cup on heat. Add beeswax and let melt.

6. Remove from heat when melted. Wait a minute or two to cool, then add essential oils and vitamin E oil. Stir to mix well.

7. Pour mixture into salve tins and allow to cool and set. Once cool, replace the lid and use as needed.

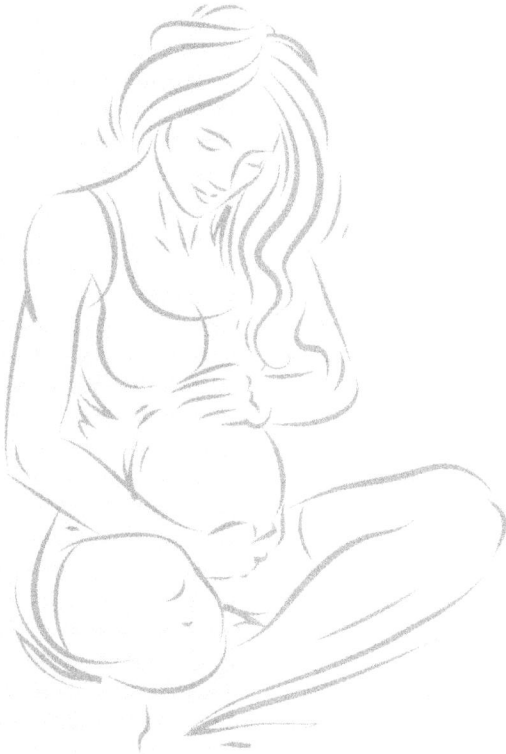

# Stretch Marks

When the skin stretches rapidly, it can lead to marks known as stretch marks. These marks could become slightly sore or itchy, and most women wish to diminish their appearance. Topical use of essential oils, via a lotion or massage oil, can help with the appearance of stretch marks. Essential oils that may help include frankincense, geranium, helichrysum, lavender, neroli, rose, Roman chamomile, and tangerine.

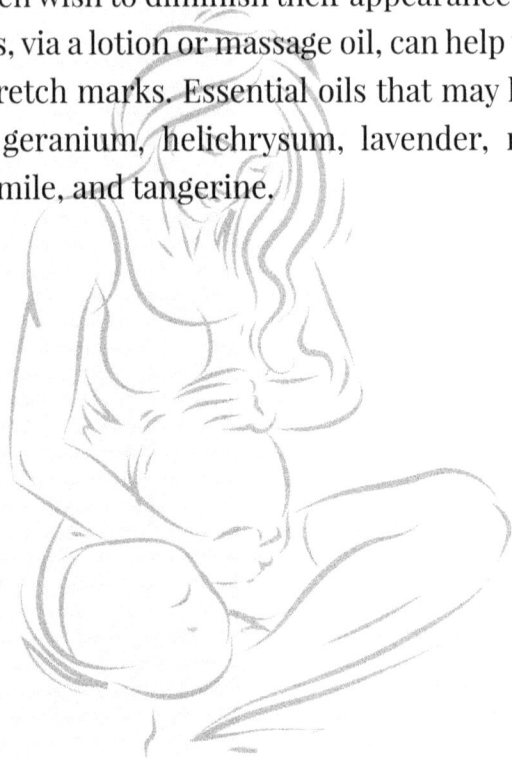

## *Stretch Mark Salve*

**What You Will Need:**

¼ cup shea butter
¼ cup coconut oil
3 tablespoons apricot kernel oil
1 tablespoon calendula flowers (optional)
¼ teaspoon dried ginger root
2 drops helichrysum essential oil
2 drops frankincense essential oil
1 drop rose essential oil (or substitute: geranium or neroli)
small glass jar with lid

**What To Do:**

1. If you are using the calendula and dried ginger, add to apricot kernel or almond oil and place in a double boiler or glass measuring cup in a small pan of water.

2. Bring to a simmer and heat for 30 minutes on medium-low heat to incorporate the properties of the herbs.

3. When the time is up, strain through a cheesecloth or metal strainer to remove herbs. You will need at least two tablespoons or more of liquid oil after straining.

4. Return the oil to the double boiler or glass measuring cup and add the shea butter and coconut oil. Heat until melted and stir as needed to blend.

5. Remove from heat and let cool for a few minutes.

6. Add essential oils and stir well. Immediately pour into a small jar or tin.

**To Use:** Rub salve on stomach, legs, and areas of concern during and after the pregnancy as needed.

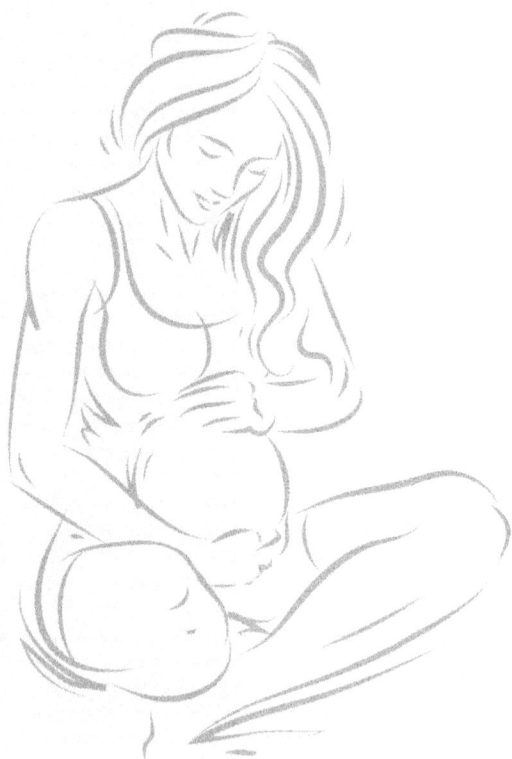

## *Stretch Mark Magic Eraser*

**What You Will Need:**

5 tablespoons rosehip seed oil
2 tablespoons moringa oil
1 teaspoon sea buckthorn seed oil
1 teaspoon vitamin E oil
1 tablespoon beeswax
2 tablespoons shea butter
12 drops helichrysum essential oil
8 drops lavender essential oil

**What To Do:**

1. Combine rosehip seed oil, moringa oil, sea buckthorn oil, vitamin E oil, beeswax, and shea butter in a glass pyrex measuring cup.

2. Set the container on canning jar rings in a medium-sized pan. Add water to the pan to the level of oils. Be careful not to get water in the measuring cup. Heat to melt together.

3. Remove from heat and let cool. Pour into a glass bottle for storage.

**To Use:** Massage oil into areas of concern and use as needed.

# Urinary Tract Infection

A urinary tract infection (UTI) is an infection in any part of your urinary system—your kidneys, ureters, bladder, and urethra. Most infections involve the lower urinary tract—the bladder and the urethra. These are common in pregnancy and should be treated as quickly as possible. Infection limited to your bladder can be painful and annoying. However, serious consequences can occur if a UTI spreads to your kidneys. Topical use over the kidneys and bladder is an efficient way of using essential oils. Essential oils that may help include cypress, grapefruit, lemon, and lime.

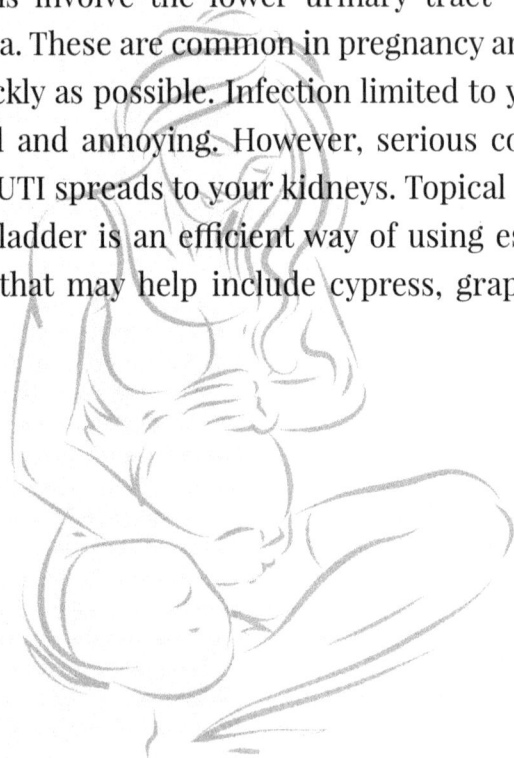

## *UTI Massage Relief*

**What You Will Need:**

10 drops juniper berry essential oil
10 drops rosemary essential oil
10 drops lemongrass essential oil
fractionated coconut oil
10 ml roller bottle

**What To Do:**

1. Remove the ball from the roller bottle and add essential oils and carrier oil.

2. Replace cap and shake to blend.

**To Use:** Roll this blend onto your tummy, lower back and over kidneys. Use twice daily.

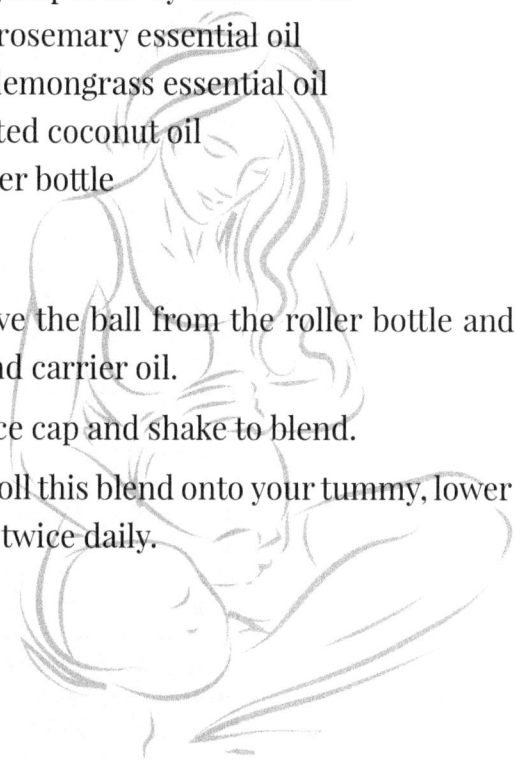

## Stop UTI Capsules

**What You Will Need:**

> 1 drop clove essential oil
> 1 drop cinnamon bark essential oil
> 1 drop lemongrass essential oil
> 1 drop rosemary essential oil
> 2 drops oregano essential oil
> 2 drops frankincense essential oil
> 1 tablespoon coconut or olive oil
> 15 ml glass bottle with cap
> glass dropper
> "00" vegetarian capsules

**What To Do:**

1. In a glass bottle, combine essential oils and carrier oil. Replace cap and shake to blend.

2. Using a glass dropper, fill the gel capsule with the blend.

**To Use:** Take one capsule twice a day for three days.

# Varicose Veins

Pregnancy can cause varicose veins to form, most commonly on the legs. Making a massage oil or lotion is an excellent way of using essential oils for varicose veins. Essential oils that may help include cypress, geranium, lemon, orange, and sandalwood.

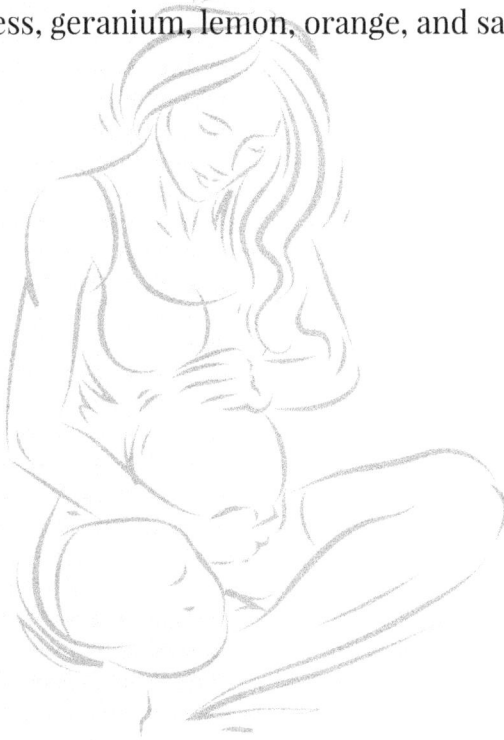

## Varicose Vein Massage Oil

**What You Will Need:**

2 drops black pepper essential oil

8 drops cypress essential oil

4 drops German chamomile essential oil

4 drops helichrysum essential oil

6 drops lemongrass essential oil

4 drops peppermint essential oil

4 drops rosemary essential oil

2 drops sandalwood essential oil

2 drops yarrow essential oil

2 ounces fractionated coconut oil (or almond oil or grapeseed oil)

2-ounce glass dropper bottle

**What To Do:**

1. In a glass bottle, add the essential oils and fill the remaining space with the carrier oil (up to the shoulder of the bottle).

2. Replace cap and shake to blend.

**To Use:** Place a nickel-sized amount of the blend in your palm and apply to the area above the varicose vein in a gentle upward motion twice a day. Allow the essential oil blend to be absorbed into the skin before getting dressed. It can take several months before seeing improvement, so be diligent in using regularly. Afterward, you can use daily thereafter for maintenance.

## *Varicose Vein Healing Balm*

**What You Will Need:**

7 tablespoons sweet almond oil

24 drops black pepper essential oil

12 drops nutmeg essential oil

1 tablespoon beeswax

4-ounce glass jar with lid

**What To Do:**

1. In a double boiler, melt the beeswax in the almond oil. Remove from heat once the beeswax melts. Stir as needed.

2. Let cool for one minute, then add essential oils.

3. Pour into a 4-ounce jar with a lid. Allow the mixture to set up overnight.

**To Use:** Apply the salve and massage into concern areas as needed.

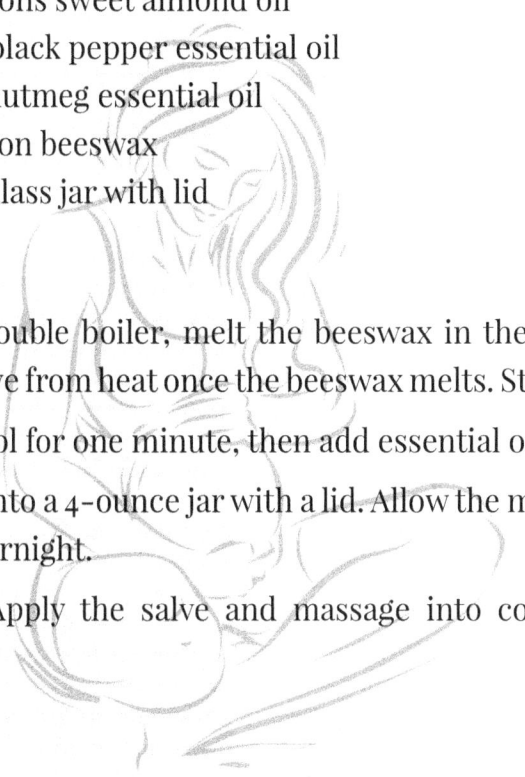

## Varicose Vein Roller Blend

**What You Will Need:**

> 5 drops cypress essential oil
>
> 3 drops helichrysum essential oil
>
> 5 drops lemongrass essential oil
>
> fractionated coconut oil (or another favorite carrier oil)
>
> 10 ml glass roller bottle

**What To Do:**

1. In a 10 ml roll-on bottle, add the essential oil and fill the remaining space with the carrier oil.

2. Replace the roller ball and the lid. Shake to blend.

**To Use:** Roll over the affected area and massage the oil in the skin. Elevate the feet afterward.

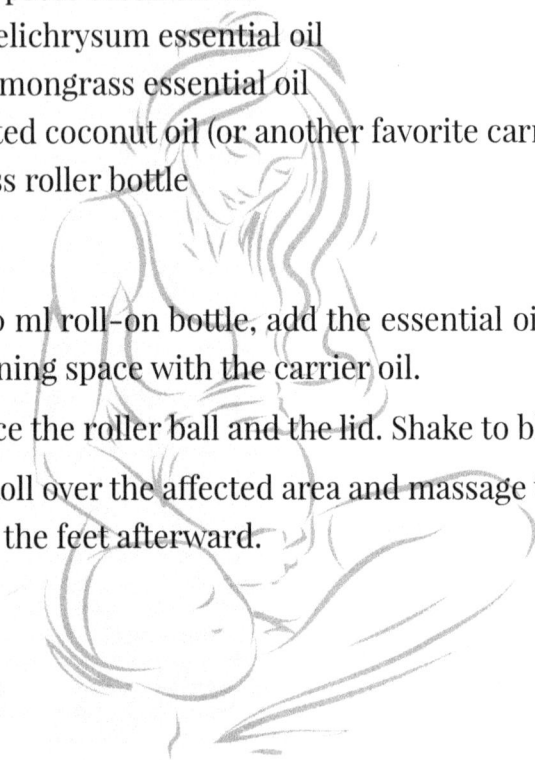

# Yeast Infection

During pregnancy, the pH of the vagina can change and allow candida to collect, which then can turn into a yeast infection. An aromatic bath, spritz, or vaginal pessary are the best ways for addressing yeast infections with essential oils. Essential oils that may help with this include bergamot, German chamomile, lavender, lemongrass, and tea tree.

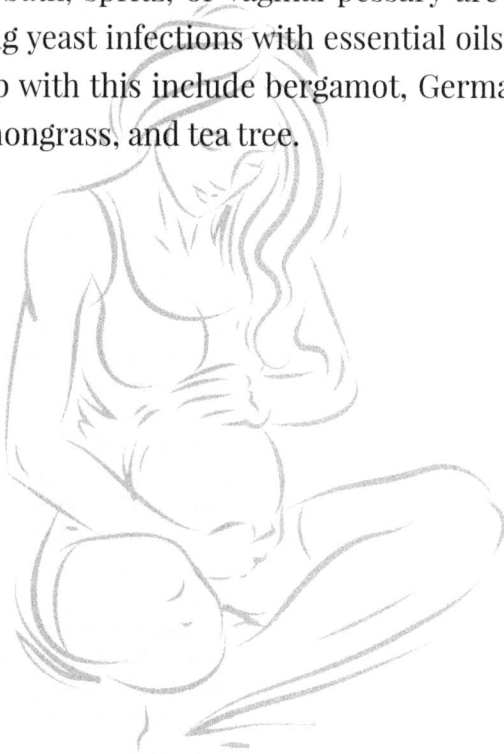

## Yeast Infection Treatment

**What You Will Need:**

2 drops lavender essential oil
2 drops tea tree essential oil
½ teaspoon raw honey
1 teaspoon plain yogurt (organic is best with no flavoring or sugar added)
2 teaspoons unrefined coconut oil
tampon (cotton, organic if possible)
pad
glass bowl

**What To Do:**

1. In a glass bowl, add the essential oils and coconut oil together.

2. Next, add the honey and yogurt in and mix well.

3. Remove the tampon from its packaging and roll in the mixture to absorb the contents.

**To Use:** Insert into the vagina before going to bed. Be sure to wear a pad in your underwear to absorb any discharge. In the morning, remove and wash off area in the shower. Repeat every night for five days.

## *Yeast Infection Treatment #2*

**What You Will Need:**

5 drops German chamomile essential oil
5 drops lavender essential oil
5 drops tea tree essential oil
4 ounces plain yogurt (with live cultures)
glass bowl
cotton tampon

**What To Do:**

1. In a glass bowl, combine yogurt and essential oils.

2. Place tampon cotton in the bowl and roll to cover with the yogurt mixture.

**To Use:** Insert tampon into the vagina before bedtime. Remove in the morning and shower to clean the area. Use once a day as needed.

## Yeast Infection Douche

**What You Will Need:**

> 2 drops lavender essential oil
> 2 drops rosemary essential oil
> 2 drops tea tree essential oil
> 2 tablespoons vinegar
> 2 ½ cups warm distilled water
> waterbottle douche kit

**What To Do:**

1. In a bowl, mix together vinegar, water, and essential oils.

2. Pour vinegar solution into the douche and irrigate your vagina once a day for three days.

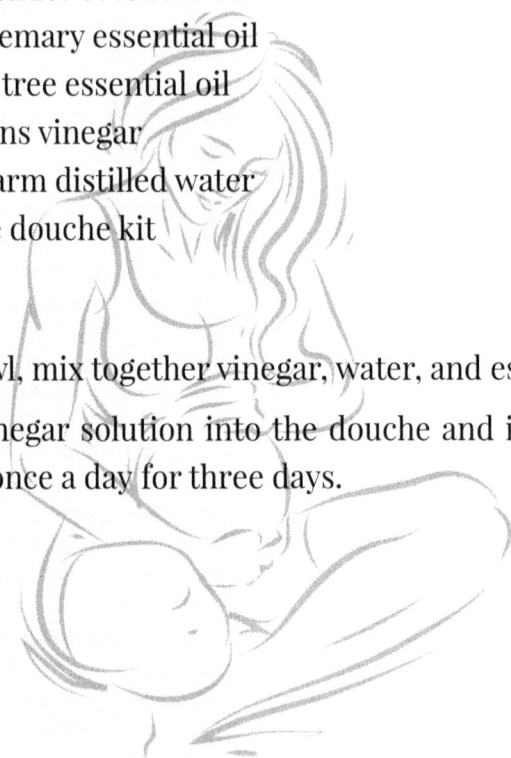

# Other Pregnancy Symptoms

Other less obvious symptoms of pregnancy that you might experience during the first trimester include:

- **Moodiness.** The flood of hormones in your body in early pregnancy can make you unusually emotional and weepy. Mood swings also are common. Oils to use: lavender and geranium.

- **Bloating.** Hormonal changes during early pregnancy can cause you to feel bloated, similar to how you might feel at the start of a menstrual period. Oils to use: ginger and peppermint.

- **Light spotting.** Sometimes a small amount of light spotting is one of the first signs of pregnancy. Known as implantation bleeding, it happens when the fertilized egg attaches to the lining of the uterus—about 10 to 14 days after conception. Implantation bleeding occurs around the time of a menstrual period. However, not all women have it. Oils to use: lavender and rose.

- **Cramping.** Some women experience mild uterine cramping early in pregnancy. Oils to use: Roman chamomile and lavender.

- **Food aversions.** When you're pregnant, you might become more sensitive to certain odors and your sense of taste might change. Like most other symptoms of pregnancy, these food preferences can be chalked up to hormonal changes. Oils to use: mandarin and lemon.

- **Nasal congestion.** Increasing hormone levels and blood

production can cause the mucous membranes in your nose to swell, dry out, and bleed easily. This might cause you to have a stuffy or runny nose. Oils to use: eucalyptus and peppermint.

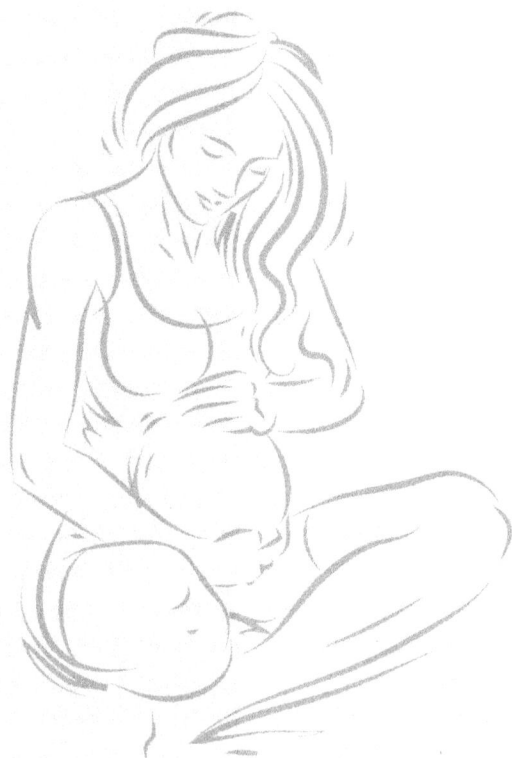

# Labor & Delivery

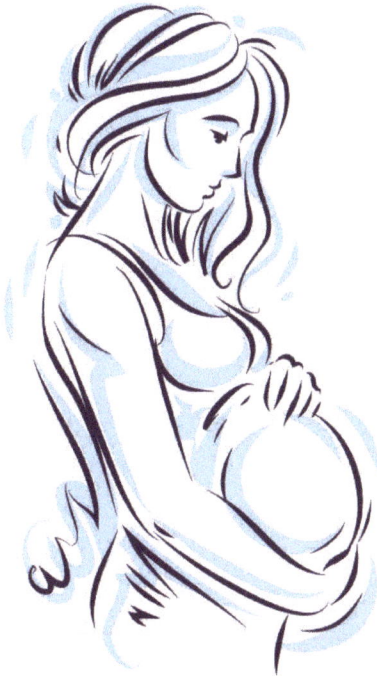

Y ou have gotten through the pregnancy, and now the big day is here—you are in labor. In this section, we're going to be talking about essential oils that can help support you through labor and delivery, and which oils you should take with you to the event.

Below are some of the common concerns during labor and delivery, which essential oils can be helpful, and how to use them. Special note about using essential oils during labor: there may be times when certain scents of essential oils become overwhelming. If this happens, it's okay, shelve the essential oils, try a different oil, or find comfort in another way during this time.

## Anxiety

Some moms may be anxious about the labor and delivery process, especially first-time moms. Even experienced moms may feel anxiety about the changing family dynamic. Aromatic use is best for anxiety. Essential oils that may help include basil, bergamot, Virginian cedarwood, Roman chamomile, cypress, frankincense, jasmine, lavender, lemon, lime, marjoram, neroli, melissa, orange, palmarosa, patchouli, rose, sandalwood, vetiver, and ylang ylang.

## *Mama's Xanax Diffuser Blend*

**What You Will Need:**

> 2 drops geranium essential oil
> 2 drops clary sage essential oil
> 1 drop patchouli essential oil
> 1 drop ylang ylang essential oil
> 15 ml glass bottle

**What To Do:**

1. Add essential oils to the water in an ultrasonic cool-mist diffuser.

2. If using a cool-air nebulizing diffuser, multiply this blend by 10 and place in a 15 ml glass bottle and run for 30 minutes to one hour before going to bed, or apply 1 to 2 drops of this blend to palms and take 3 to 5 deep belly breaths.

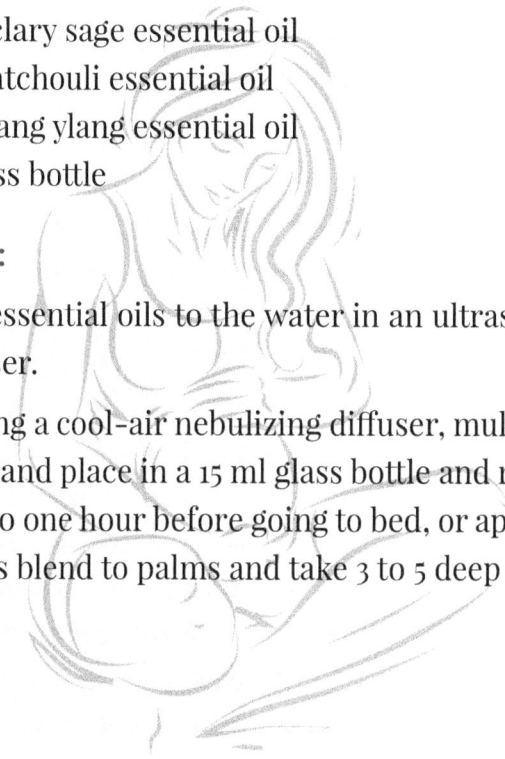

## *Chill Pill Diffuser Blend*

**What You Will Need:**

> 20 drops cedarwood essential oil
> 20 drops wild orange essential oil
> 10 drops ylang ylang essential oil
> 10 drops patchouli essential oil
> 15 ml glass bottle

**What To Do:**

1. Add essential oils to a glass bottle, replace the cap, and shake to blend.

2. Store until ready to use.

**To Use:** Add several drops of the essential oil blend into an ultrasonic cool-air diffuser. If using a cool-air nebulizing diffuser, place glass bottle into the diffuser and run for 30 minutes to one hour before going to bed.

## *Bedtime Diffuser Blend*

**What You Will Need:**

> 2 drops clary sage essential oil
> 2 drops lavender essential oil
> 1 drop bergamot essential oil

**What To Do:**

1. Add the essential oils to a water-based ultrasonic diffuser.

2. If you are using a cool-air nebulizing diffuser, multiply this blend by 10 in a 15 ml glass bottle and run for 30 minutes to one hour before going to bed.

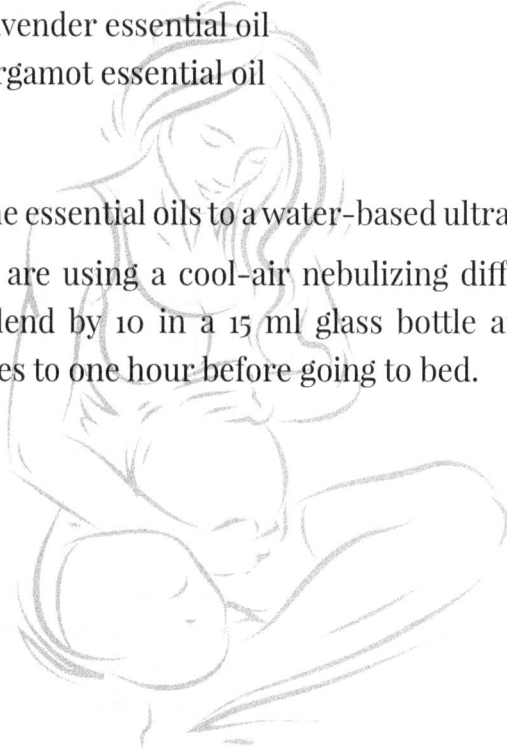

# Back Labor

The pain and discomfort experienced in the lower back during labor—occurs in about 25 percent of women. Uterine contractions cause both regular and back labor contractions. But with back labor, your baby is usually in the "sunny-side up" position. That means your baby's little head is down by your cervix, but he's facing your stomach instead of your back. This is common in labor and delivery—instead of feeling contractions in front, a woman feels them in their back, and they can be quite intense. A topical blend massaged into the back can be very helpful for this. Essential oils that may help include black pepper, cajeput, German chamomile, cinnamon bark, eucalyptus, ginger, juniper berry, lavender, lemon, marjoram, nutmeg, peppermint, pine, and rosemary.

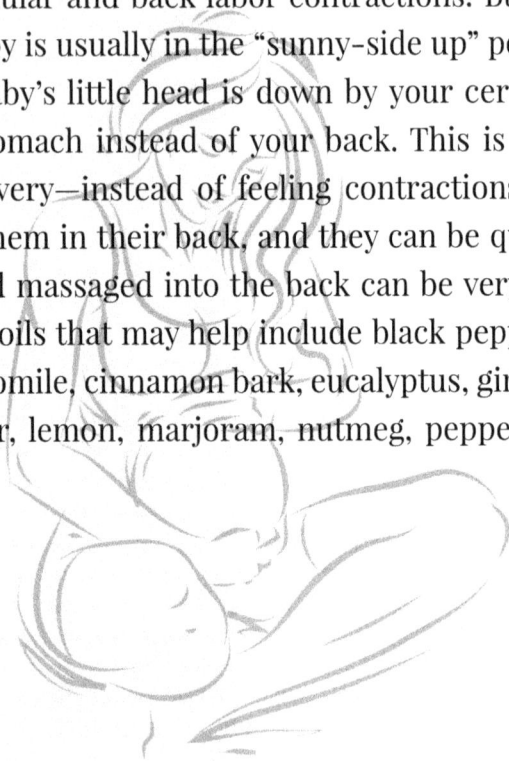

## *Backpain Labor Salve*

**What You Will Need:**

4 drops black pepper essential oil
4 drops peppermint essential oil
1 ounce shea butter
1-ounce glass jar
glass pyrex measuring cup

**What To Do:**

1.  In a pyrex measuring cup or double boiler, melt the shea butter. Once it is completely melted, remove from heat.

2.  After allowing to cool one minute, add the essential oils. Stir well and store in a cool, dark place.

**To Use:** Take this cream with you in your labor bag to have as a salve for any muscle pain you are experiencing during labor. This blend is also useful for tight shoulders.

## Backpain Labor Diffuser Blend

**What You Will Need:**

3 drops orange essential oil

3 drops peppermint essential oil

2 drops geranium essential oil

**What To Do:**

1. Add the essential oils to a water-based ultrasonic diffuser (if the hospital allows).

2. If a diffuser is not allowed, use the blend in an aromatherapy inhaler. Even in a short labor, this blend could be helpful around transition when labor is most intense and pushing will come soon.

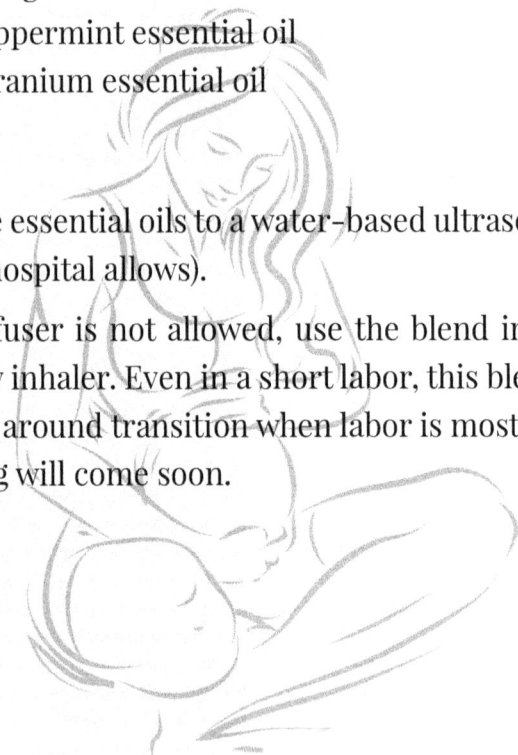

# Mastitis

Mastitis is an inflammation of breast tissue that sometimes involves an infection. It occurs when the milk ducts become blocked and inflamed. This can lead to painful swelling and breast engorgement, warmth, and redness. You might also have fever and chills. Mastitis most commonly affects women who are breast-feeding (lactation mastitis). Lactation mastitis can cause you to feel run down, making it difficult to care for your baby. Sometimes mastitis leads a mother to wean her baby before she intends to. Applying essential oils topically works best for this condition. Essential oils that may help include clary sage, geranium, helichrysum, lavender, neroli, and rose.

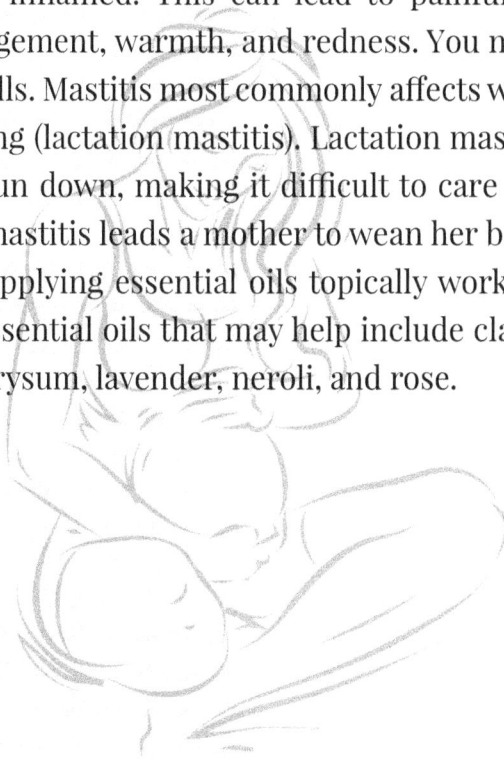

## Mastitis Massage Oil

**What You Will Need:**

> 3 drops tea tree essential oil
> 3 drops lavender essential oil
> 3 drops roman chamomile essential oil
> 1 tablespoon fractionated coconut oil
> 15 ml glass bottle

**What To Do:**

1. Add essential oils and coconut oil to a glass bottle.

2. Replace lid and shake to blend.

**To Use:** Gently massage into the sides of the breast and under both armpits.

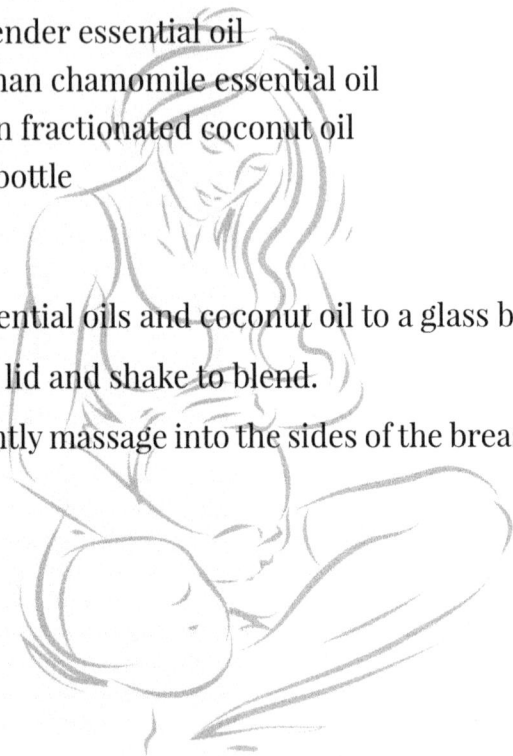

## *Boob Job Salve*

**What You Will Need:**

8 ounces olive oil
8 ounces fresh comfrey leaves
1 ounce beeswax
10 drops peppermint essential oil
10 drops tea tree essential oil
10 drops eucalyptus essential oil
10 drops lavender essential oil
1 tablespoon vitamin E oil
glass measuring cup

**What To Do:**

1. Chop or tear comfrey leaves into small pieces and place in a glass measuring cup. Cover them with the olive oil.

2. Place measuring cup with oil and comfrey leaves in a pan of water over medium heat (140 degrees F). Keep it at this temperature for about 3 ½ hours.

3. Remove from heat. Strain the oil, removing the leaves.

4. Add the beeswax to the oil and place back in the double boiler or pan of water to melt the beeswax. Stir the mixture continually until completely melted.

5. After the beeswax is melted, remove from heat. Add the essential oils and vitamin E oil. Stir to blend well.

6. Pour the liquid salve into a 2-ounce canning jar or small metal container with lids. Set the container aside without the lid on to allow the salve to harden.

**To Use:** Apply around breasts and under armpits two times a day. Be sure to clean breasts before nursing.

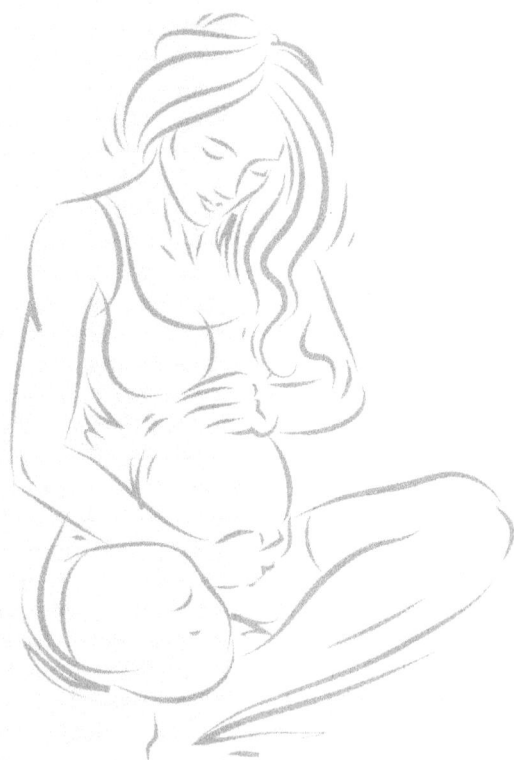

# Blood Pressure

Blood pressure can rise and fall during pregnancy and the post-partum period. Using essential oils aromatically can help, with the main focus being on helping mom to relax to keep her blood pressure down. Essential oils that may help include bergamot, Roman chamomile, clary sage, helichrysum, lavender, lemon, orange, neroli, and rose.

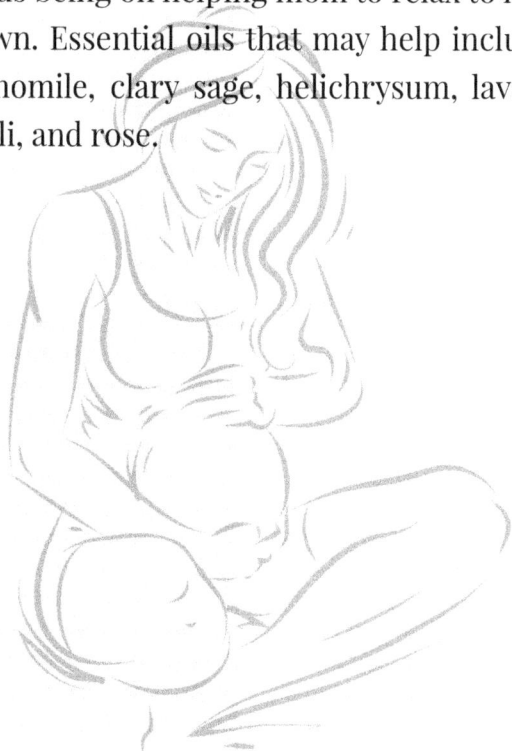

## *Lower BP Massage Oil*

**What You Will Need:**

> 5 drops lavender essential oil
> 5 drops clary sage essential oil
> 5 drops frankincense essential oil
> 2 ounces fractionated coconut oil
> 2-ounce glass bottle

**What To Do:**

1.  In a glass bottle, add essential oils and coconut oil (or another carrier oil).

2.  Replace lid and shake to blend.

**To Use:** Take a nickel-sized amount into your palm and rub into your neck, temples, and upper chest area. Use as needed.

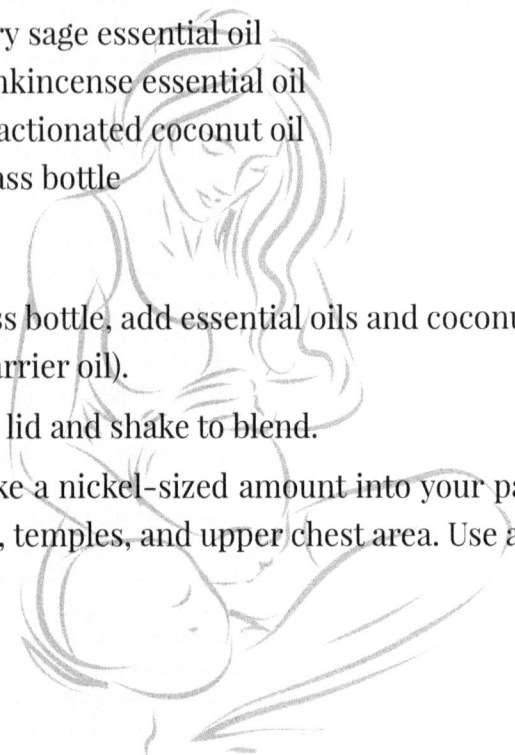

## BP Diffuser Blend

**What You Will Need:**

> 3 drops bergamot essential oil
> 3 drops lavender essential oil
> 3 drops ylang ylang essential oil

**What To Do:**

1. Add the essential oils into a water-based ultrasonic diffuser or add oils to an aromatherapy inhaler.

2. Run the diffuser for 15 to 20 minutes.

**To Use:** Slowly breathe in and inhale the oils to help lower your blood pressure.

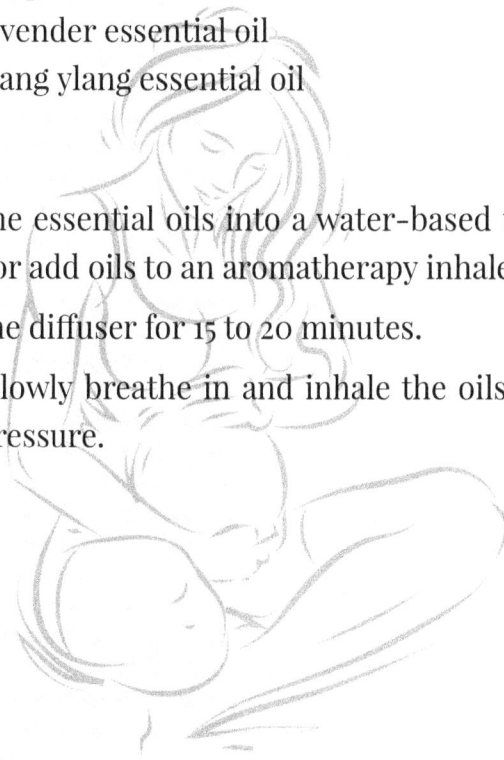

## BP Roll-On

**What You Will Need:**

4 drops lavender essential oil

2 drops ylang ylang essential oil

3 drops marjoram essential oil

1 drop neroli essential oil

2 teaspoons almond oil

roll-on bottle

**What To Do:**

1. Remove the ball from the bottle and add essential oils. Fill the remaining space with the carrier oil.

2. Replace ball and lid. Shake to blend.

**To Use:** Roll oils over carotid arteries and wrists. Use as needed several times a day.

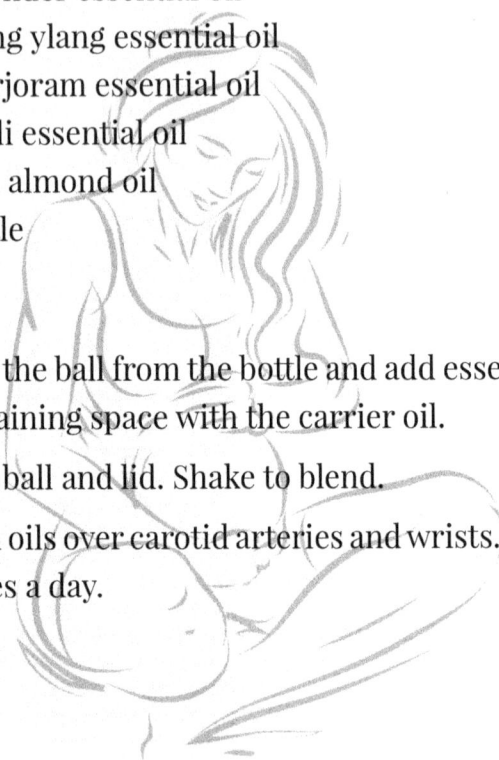

# Childbirth Pain

Pain is an inevitable part of giving birth to a child. Contractions are painful, and it will get more intense as the labor progresses. Transitioning is generally touted as one of the most painful times of the process. Thankfully, aromatic support can help with pain relief. The oils for pain during labor are listed, but let's dive a little deeper into how to use these oils to help decrease pain.

## *Diffuser*

Diffusing oils can help mom's pain perception and lead her to feel less pain. Beneficial oils for relaxing include lavender, clary sage, bergamot, and orange. In the case that a diffuser is not allowed in the hospital, create a personal inhaler or aromatic room spray ahead of time for this.

## *Bath Oil*

A warm bath can go a long way in alleviating pain during labor. The warmth of the water helps to relax the muscles and can ease the pain of contractions. Using an aromatic bath oil can increase these effects. Oils such as lavender, clary sage, jasmine, geranium, and rose can be of great help here.

## *Massage Oil*

A massage oil can be applied to the mom's uterus or her lower back to help with pain control. Sweet almond oil or jojoba oil are great options for carrier oils, and clary sage, geranium, jasmine, cypress, frankincense, lavender, and rose are all great essential oil options.

# Contractions

Contractions occurs when the muscles around the uterus tighten and relax. They can occur at any time throughout pregnancy. But "real" contractions only occur when labor is starting. Real labor contractions can be painful, and the pain will intensify. It usually peaks when the muscles tighten and ease when they relax. The location of the pain varies, but real contractions typically cause a dull ache around the abdomen and lower back. In some women, the pain spreads to the sides and thighs. Labor typically starts with regular, persistent contractions. These cause the cervix to expand in preparation for birth. You can help keep contractions steady and aid in pain relief by using essential oils topically or aromatically. If using topically, apply over the area of the uterus. Essential oils that may help include black pepper, clary sage, geranium, jasmine, marjoram, and neroli.

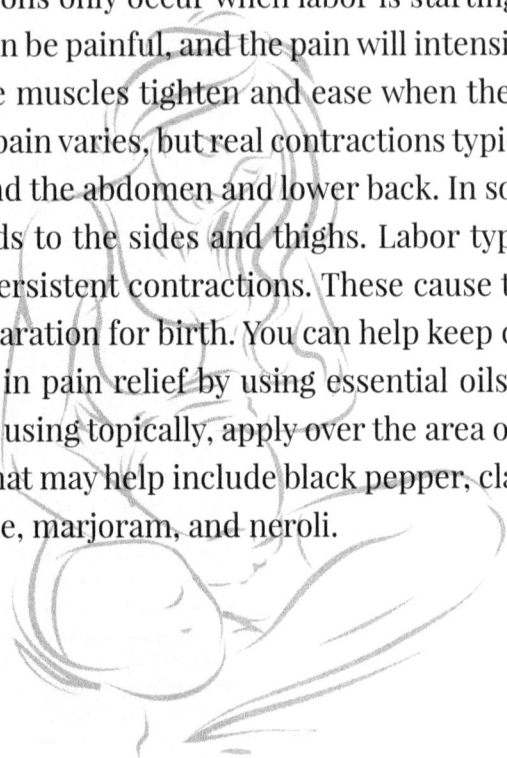

## *Labor Support Blend*

**What You Will Need:**

6 drops black pepper essential oil
8 drops neroli essential oil
6 drops jasmine essential oil
30 ml fractionated coconut oil
1-ounce glass bottle

**What To Do:**

1.  In a glass bottle, add the essential oils and fill the remaining space with the carrier oil.

2.  Shake to mix oils.

**To Use:** Massage into abdomen and back before or during labor to promote contractions and relaxation.

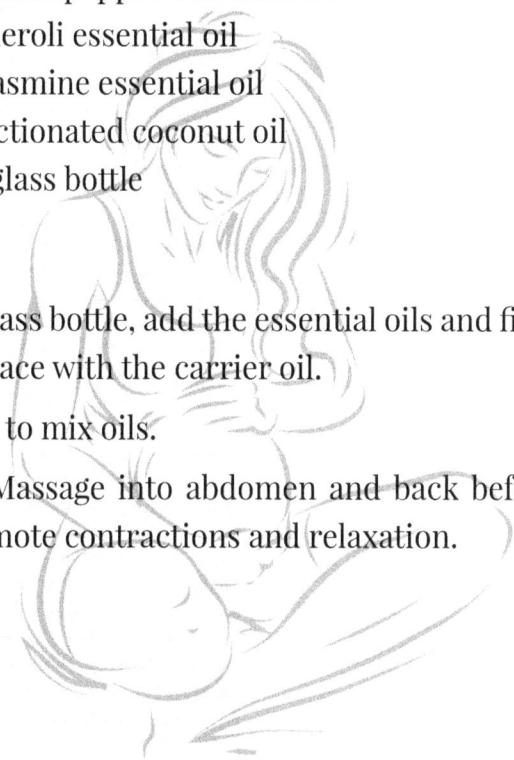

# Labor Progression

Sometimes, labor slows down or stalls out. You can help get things going by applying essential oils over the uterus and using them aromatically. Essential oils that may help include clary sage, fennel, lavender, jasmine, neroli, and rose.

## *Rose and Clary Sage Oil Blend*

**What You Will Need:**

> 2 drops rose essential oil
> 2 drops clary sage essential oil
> 1 teaspoon sweet almond oil

**What To Do:**

1.  Place a teaspoon of almond oil in your palm.

2.  Add essential oils and stir with finger to blend.

**To Use:** Apply the blend on the tummy to assist with encouraging contractions.

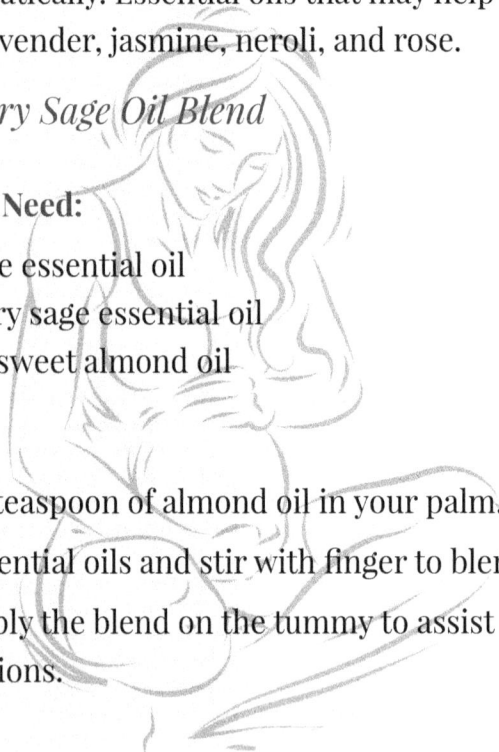

## *Lavender Oil Blend*

**What You Will Need:**

2 drops lavender essential oil
1 drop Roman chamomile essential oil
1 teaspoon shea butter

**What To Do:**

1. Place a small amount of shea butter into your hand. Add essential oils.

2. Stir with finger to blend.

**To Use:** Apply as needed to help with labor.

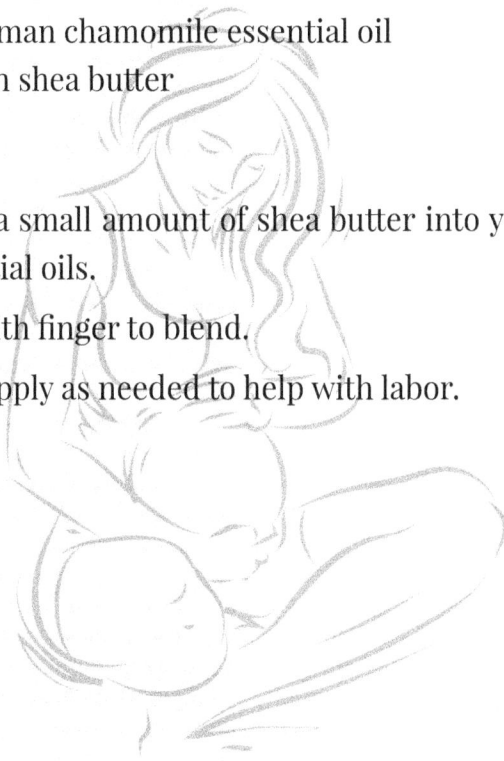

## *Peppermint Oil Blend*

**What You Will Need:**

1 drop peppermint essential oil

1 drop Roman chamomile essential oil

1 drop frankincense essential oil

1 teaspoon coconut oil

**What To Do:**

1. Pour a small amount of coconut oil into your palm. Add the essential oils.

2. Mix oils together with your finger.

**To Use:** Apply the blend over abdomen and back.

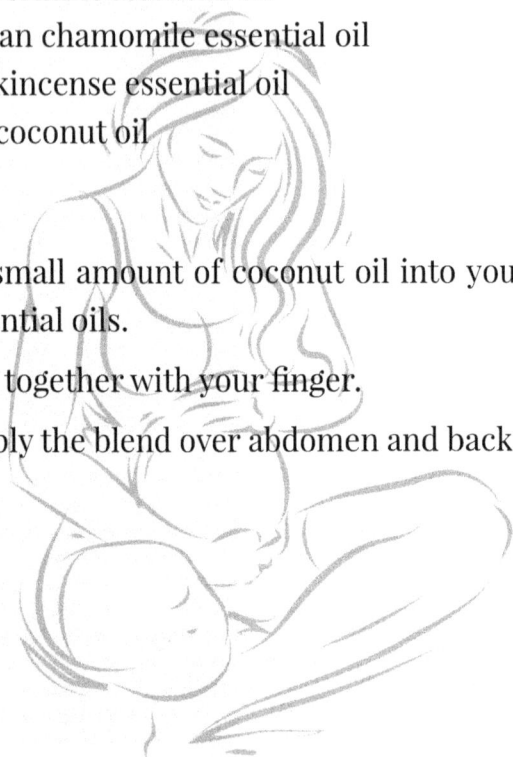

## Transition

During the transition, mom may find herself feeling exhausted, anxious, and in an increased amount of pain. Applying essential oils over the abdomen (see the section for contractions for essential oils to use) can help with the pain, while using oils aromatically can help with the fear and exhaustion. Essential oils that may help include bergamot, clary sage, grapefruit, jasmine, lemon, lime, mandarin, orange, patchouli, rose, rosemary, and spearmint.

## *Transition Lotion*

**What You Will Need:**

10 drops mandarin essential oil

5 drops grapefruit essential oil

5 drops jasmine essential oil

5 drops rosemary essential oil

5 drops spearmint essential oil

2 ounces unscented lotion

2-ounce bottle or glass bottle with a pump top

**What To Do:**

1. In a squeeze-top or pump bottle, add lotion.

2. Add essential oils to the lotion and stir to blend well.

**To Use:** Apply as needed over the abdomen to help with the pain.

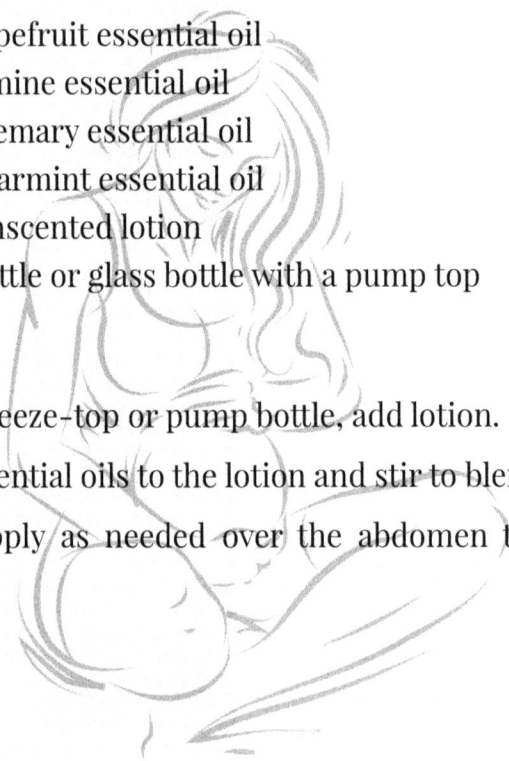

## *Transition Diffuser Blend*

**What You Will Need:**

12 drops bergamot essential oil
6 drops rose essential oil
3 drops lime essential oil
3 drops patchouli essential oil
5 ml glass bottle

**What To Do:**

1. In a 5 ml glass bottle, add essential oils.

2. Replace cap and shake to blend.

**To Use:** Place 6-8 drops of your essential oil blend into your diffuser. You can also use this blend for a personal inhaler as well if a diffuser is not allowed in the hospital.

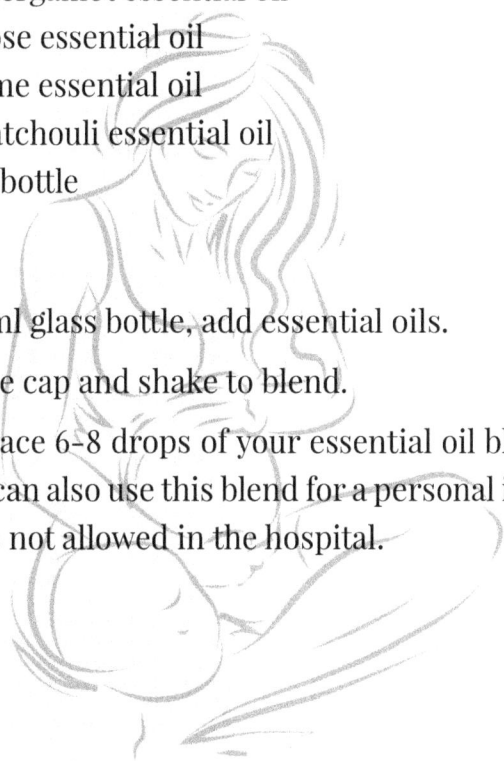

# Muscle Tension

Labor is hard work and can lead to tense and sore muscles. A massage oil or lotion applied topically can help to alleviate these symptoms. Essential oils that may help include basil, black pepper, cypress, lavender, marjoram, and peppermint.

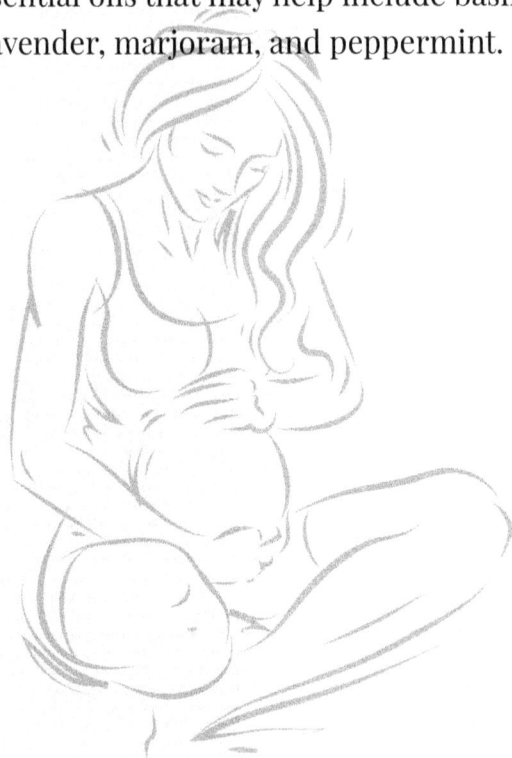

## *Pain Away Massage Oil*

**What You Will Need:**

>  10 drops cypress essential oil
>  5 drops basil essential oil
>  5 drops lavender essential oil
>  5 drops black pepper essential oil
>  10 drops marjoram essential oil
>  60 ml grapeseed oil (or another favorite carrier oil)
>  2-ounce dark glass bottle

**What To Do:**

1.  In a glass bottle, add the essential oils and carrier oil.

2.  Replace cap and shake to blend.

**To Use:** Have your spouse or birth support partner massage the essential oil blend into your belly or lower back during contractions.

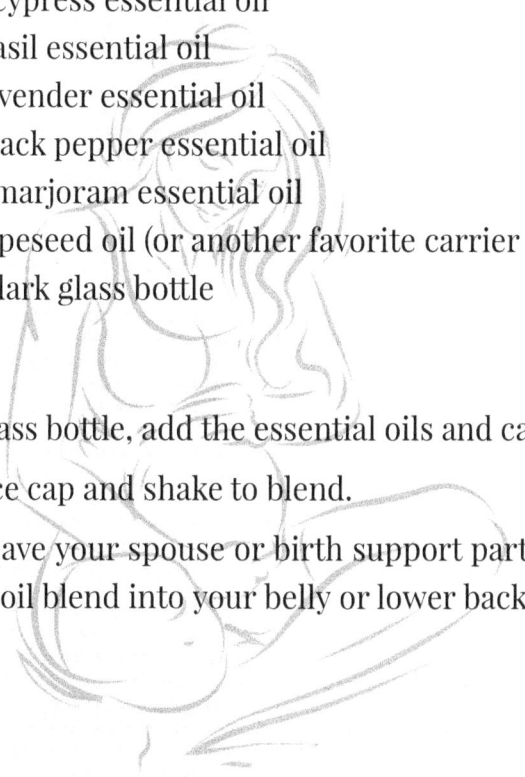

# Perineal Care

The perineum needs care after natural childbirth—it can become infected or just be sore and bruised. A gentle, soothing spray can be helpful for this condition. Essential oils that may help include frankincense, helichrysum, lavender, and tea tree. Hydrosols that may be helpful include: lavender, tea tree, helichrysum, and calendula.

# C-Section Wound Care

Even with the best-laid birth plan, things don't always go accordingly, and sometimes a c-section is necessary. While aromatic support probably won't be allowed to continue in the operating room, you can use aromatics afterward for wound care. Applying the oils topically in a salve or spritz can be helpful. Essential oils that may help include frankincense, helichrysum, lavender, and tea tree. Hydrosols that might be helpful include: calendula, lavender, helichrysum, and tea tree.

The days following the birth of your baby, the postpartum period, can be one of the most challenging times for mothers and families. This period can be even more challenging for mothers who have had a cesarean delivery. After any delivery, a mother needs to allow her body to rest and heal. Ideally, this means little to no housework, and no running after other little ones.

During this time, special consideration needs to be given to the care of the mother. If you are a single mother or your partner has to return to work shortly after the birth of the child, try to organize a support team prior to the birth of your child to help during this time.

## C-Section Gel

**What You Will Need:**

> 1 ounce aloe vera gel
> 3 drops tea tree essential oil
> 3 drops frankincense essential oil
> 3 drops lavender essential oil
> cotton pad

**What To Do:**

1.  In a glass bowl, add aloe vera gel and essential oils together. Apply to the incision area and allow the gel to dry.

2.  Cover area with a cotton pad to keep it dry and absorb any oozing that may come from the affected area. If your healthcare provider recommends that you not dress the wound, you can apply the gel and leave it uncovered to encourage faster healing. If your skin reacts negatively to the essential oils, stop use immediately.

## C-Section Salve

**What You Will Need:**

10 drops lavender essential oil

10 drops frankincense essential oil

10 drops geranium essential oil

10 drops German chamomile essential oil

10 drops tea tree essential oil

1 cup coconut oil

1 teaspoon vitamin E oil

glass jar

**What To Do:**

1. Place coconut oil in a bowl and use a hand mixer to whip it up. Add vitamin E oil and mix.

2. Add the essential oils to the whipped coconut oil and blend well.

3. Store the salve in a glass jar.

**To Use:** Rub over the abdomen as needed.

# Episiotomy Care

Having an episiotomy, or tearing, can be painful for mom. An episiotomy is a surgical incision in the perineum (the area between the vagina and anus) made just before delivery to enlarge the vaginal opening. After the baby is delivered, stitches will be used to close the incision or any tears that occur accidentally during delivery. Caring for these stitches is important as it helps minimize the risk of pain and infection during the postpartum healing process.

An aromatic spritzer would be great for this concern. Essential oils that may help include frankincense, helichrysum, lavender, tea tree, and petitgrain. Hydrosols that might be helpful include: calendula, helichrysum, lavender, and tea tree.

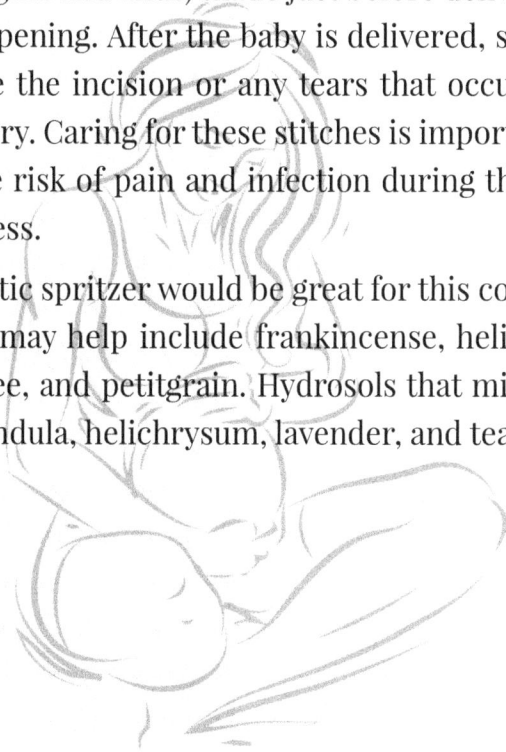

## *Episiotomy Healing Salve*

**What You Will Need:**

45 ml calendula oil

10 grams beeswax pellets

5 drops tea tree essential oil

5 drops lavender essential oil

5 drops helichrysum essential oil

pyrex glass measuring cup

sterile pad

**What To Do:**

1. In a double boiler, melt the beeswax and calendula oil together over medium heat. This can also be done in a microwave at a low setting.

2. Remove oil mixture from heat and add the essential oil. Stir with a clean spoon to mix well.

3. Pour mixture into small tins or jars.

4. Leave to cool. Once cooled and hardened, replace the lid.

**To Use:** Wash your hands and perineum thoroughly and dry it with a clean tissue before using the ointment. Gently apply ointment to the area where stitches are using a sterile pad — apply every morning and every evening for 7-10 days.

## *Episio Healing Spray*

**What You Will Need:**

6 tablespoons witch hazel

2 tablespoons aloe vera gel

2 tablespoons distilled or filtered water

5 drops lavender essential oil

5 drops frankincense essential oil

5 drops clary sage essential oil

spray bottle

**What To Do:**

1. In a small spray bottle, add all of the ingredients.

2. Replace sprayer top and shake to mix.

3. Store in refrigerator to add extra cooling relief and maintain freshness. Use within a month.

**To Use:** After childbirth to help soothe postpartum pain, spray on perineum a few times per day or on a natural pad.

# Exhaustion

Labor and delivery is an energy-intensive process. Moms-to-be may not be able to rest during the process due to the pain of contractions, and if delivering in a hospital, she may not be able to eat or drink to help keep her energy up. Aromatics can help mom stave off exhaustion and stay focused on the task at hand. The aromatic use of the essential oils, either by a diffuser, personal inhaler, or fragrant room spray, can be quite beneficial. Bright essential oils such as grapefruit, bergamot, orange, lemon, lime, and spearmint are all tremendous essential oil options.

# Enhancing the Birth Experience

When using essential oils during the labor and delivery of your child, take these steps into consideration to fully enhance your birthing experience.

1. Always use scents you like—never the ones you have an aversion to, especially for inhaling or diffusing.

2. Remember to have someone with you to support you during this emotional time. Let them know which oil you'd like to diffuse or use.

3. Be flexible—things can change in an instant, and the easier you're able to adapt, the better.

4. Be prepared—certain scents might be fine for a while, then suddenly become bothersome or stop working for pain. Bring other oils with you to switch out with the ones you were using.

5. As you begin to get closer to transition, have your part-

ner prepare which oils to use to support you when the time comes.

## Delivery Hospital Kit

1.  Create a birth kit with all of the essential oils and supplies you'll need during labor and delivery.

2.  Spend time getting familiar with the oils before the big day. Take time to educate yourself on their benefits, limitations, and proper usage.

3.  If the mom-to-be is going to be delivering in the hospital setting, be sure to check with hospital staff and doctors about essential oil use—make sure you have permission to use aromatics in their facility. Some facilities have rules that don't allow you to use a diffuser.

Provide information on aromatics to labor and delivery nurses and doctors—educating them is a good way of getting them more on board with what you plan to be using.

# Essential Oils and Supplies for Your Labor Kit

A lot of essential oils have been mentioned so far, and you can't possibly take all of them with you for your labor and delivery. So, which ones should you take? The following list is the recommended essential oils for your labor kit. Feel free to add a few others if you have favorites you want to take.

**Essential Oils:**

Bergamot
Clary Sage
Geranium
Tea Tree
Lavender
Roman Chamomile
Jasmine
Rose
Frankincense
Black Pepper
Orange
Spearmint

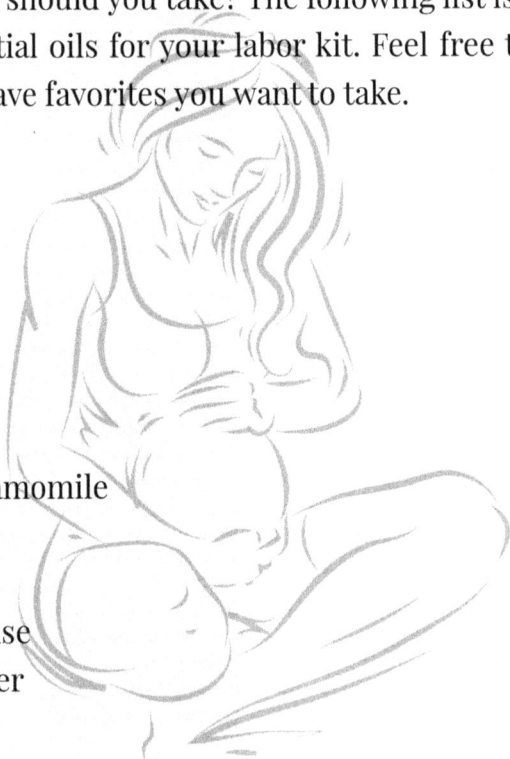

**Other Items:**

Inhalers
Empty bottles
Spray bottle filled with distilled water
Carrier oil (your choice)

# Mommy Care

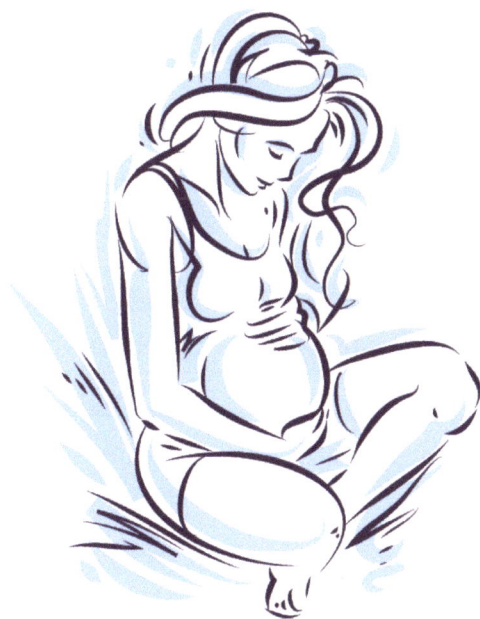

aking care of yourself and your new baby after the birth is an integral part of the process, and there are, of course, aromatic remedies that can be used. In this chapter, we will cover some of the needed care during postpartum, which essential oils can help, and how to use them.

## Breastfeeding

**Breastfeeding** is the most natural way to feed your baby. It provides all the nutrition your baby needs during the first six months of life, satisfying their hunger and thirst at the same time. It also helps to create a loving bond between you and your baby.

Breast milk has many health benefits for your baby:

- Breast milk contains all the nutrients your baby needs for the first six months
- It satisfies the baby's thirst
- It helps develop the eyes, brain, and other body systems
- The act of breastfeeding helps with jaw development
- It helps the baby resist infection and disease, even later in life
- It reduces the risk of obesity in childhood and later in life
- It contains a range of factors that protect your baby while their immune system is still developing

# Sore Breasts

Tender, swollen breasts can occur early in pregnancy due to hormonal changes which might make your breasts sensitive and sore. The discomfort will likely decrease after a few weeks as your body adjusts to hormonal changes. As your pregnancy produces more and more estrogen and progesterone, these hormones start to make changes in your body to support the baby's growth. Your breasts may feel tender and appear bigger due to increased blood flow. Your nipples might hurt and the veins might look darker under the skin. The degree of soreness, and where and how it is felt, differs for each woman. It might be sharp, stabbing, dull, throbbing, or aching. It might be felt in all or part of the breasts, one breast or both. It can also affect the armpit area. For many women, the soreness is barely noticeable. For others, the pain is so great that it affects their everyday lives. Usually, the condition goes away in time. Using essential oils topically can help with this—be sure mom washes off the essential oils prior to nursing. Essential oils that may help include Roman chamomile, cypress, geranium, and lavender.

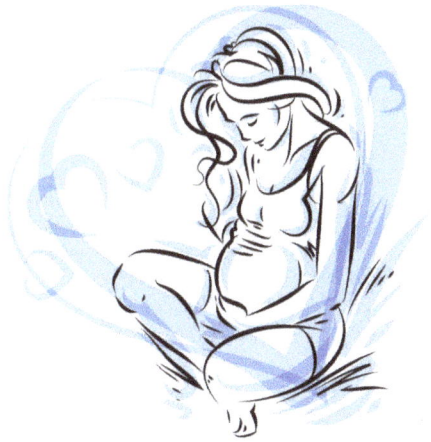

## Sore Breasts Salve

**What You Will Need:**

¼ cup coconut oil
¼ cup olive oil
1 tablespoon beeswax
12 drops lavender essential oil
4 drops geranium essential oil
4 drops Roman chamomile essential oil
4 drops cypress essential oil
4-ounce empty glass jar
small pan
stir rod

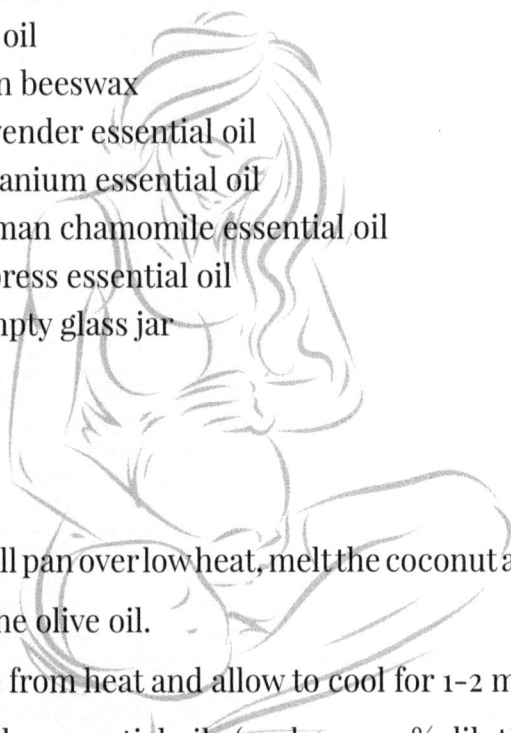

**What To Do:**

1.   In a small pan over low heat, melt the coconut and beeswax.

2.   Stir in the olive oil.

3.   Remove from heat and allow to cool for 1-2 minutes.

4.   Add in the essential oils (24 drops = 1% dilution) and mix thoroughly.

5.   Pour into a glass jar and place in the freezer to cool for 20 minutes.

6.   Replace lid and store in a cool place.

**To Use:** Apply a small amount over the breasts and nipples and massage in as needed — Wash salve off prior to nursing.

# Cracked/Dry Nipples

This can be quite painful for mom, and a nourishing cream or oil serum can be quite beneficial. Be sure to wash off the oils prior to nursing the baby. Essential oils that may help include Roman chamomile, geranium, helichrysum, lavender, and rose.

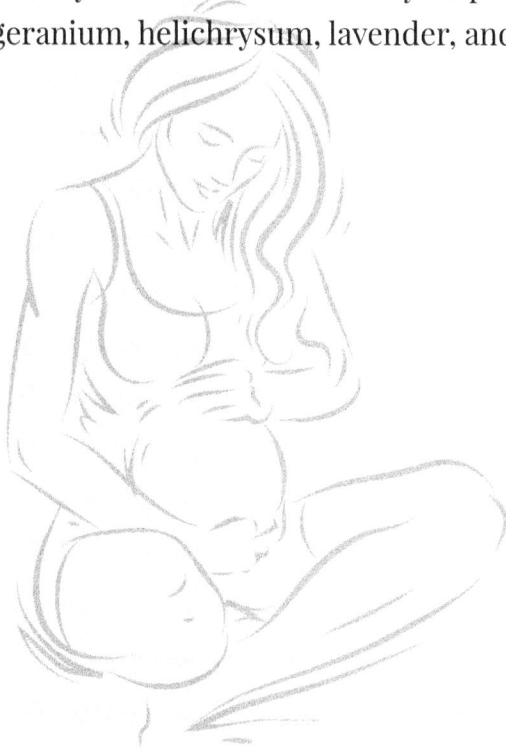

## Cracked Nipples Salve

**What You Will Need:**

2 ½ ounces shea butter
1 ounce argan oil
½ ounce avocado oil
½ ounce coconut oil
12 drops helichrysum essential oil
6 drops Roman chamomile essential oil
6 drops lavender essential oil
6 drops geranium essential oil
6 drops rose essential oil
½ ounce vitamin E oil
tin containers

**What To Do:**

1. In a double boiler, all of the ingredients and melt over medium heat.

2. Remove from heat and allow to cool for one minute. Add essential oils and stir well.

3. Pour melted mixture into 2-ounce tin containers. Allow to harden before use.

**To Use:** Apply after breastfeeding around the nipples and sore areas. Be sure to wash and remove before nursing.

## *Tender Boobs Roll-On*

**What You Will Need:**

1 ounce tamanu oil
3 drops lavender essential oil
5 drops frankincense essential oil
4 drops palmarosa essential oil
glass roller bottle

**What To Do:**

1. Remove the ball from roller bottle. Add essential oils and carrier oil.

2. Replace ball and cap and shake to blend well. Apply as needed.

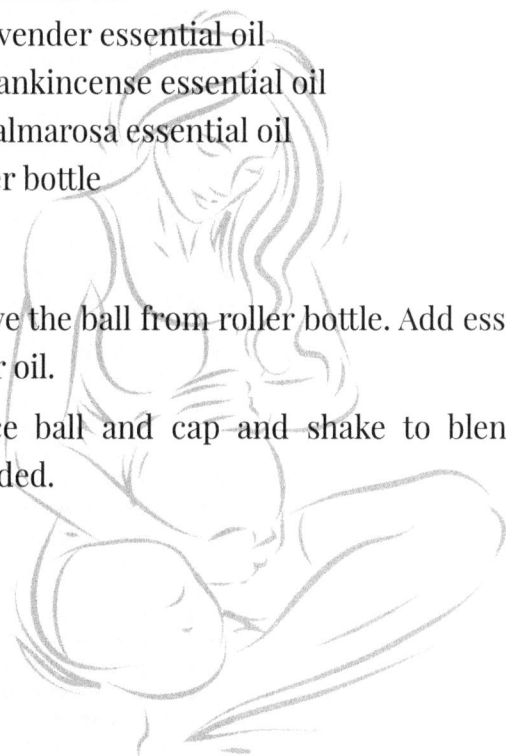

## *Hemp Oil Blend*

**What You Will Need:**

1 ounce hemp oil
7 drops palmarosa essential oil
3 drops bay laurel essential oil
5 drops lemon eucalyptus essential oil
1-ounce bottle

**What To Do:**

1. In a bottle, add hemp oil and essential oils.

2. Replace cap and shake to blend. Use as needed.

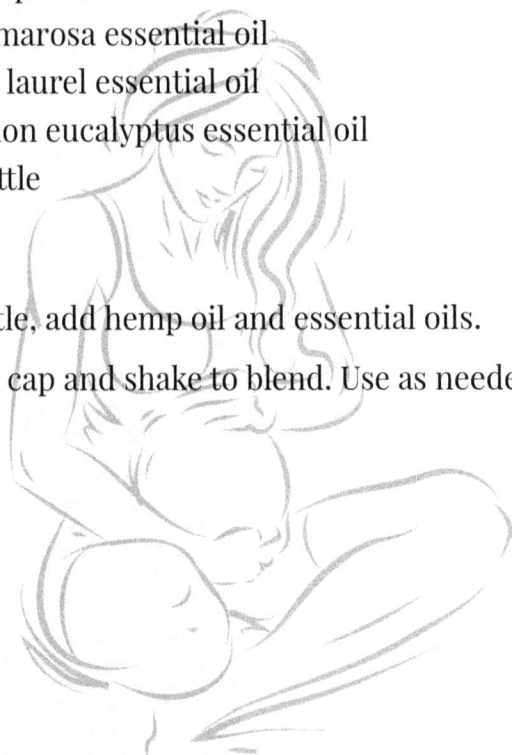

# Milk Production/Increase Lactation

Sometimes mom needs a little help getting her milk supply to increase, and using essential oils topically can help with this. However, oftentimes mothers think that their milk supply is low when it isn't. If your baby is gaining weight well on breast milk alone, then you do not have a problem with milk supply. It's important to note that the feel of the breast, the behavior of your baby, the frequency of nursing, the sensation of let-down, or the amount you pump are not valid ways to determine if you have enough milk for your baby. Using essential oils topically or aromatically can help with this. Note: the essential oils should be washed off thoroughly before nursing. Essential oils that may help include clary sage, fennel, geranium, and rose.

**Note:** Peppermint essential oil may decrease milk supply, so it is recommended to avoid this oil if breastfeeding. However, using fennel essential oil can assist in increasing mom's milk supply, and drinking fennel tea can help boost milk production.

## Milk Production Blend

**What You Will Need:**

2 drops fennel essential oil
4 drops clary sage essential oil
1 tablespoon fractionated coconut oil
10 ml glass roller bottle

**What To Do:**

1. Remove the ball from roller bottle, add essential oils, and fill the remaining space with coconut oil.

2. Replace ball and cap and shake to mix thoroughly.

**To Use:** Apply to breast, excluding nipple area, after nursing (to encourage milk flow for next feeding).

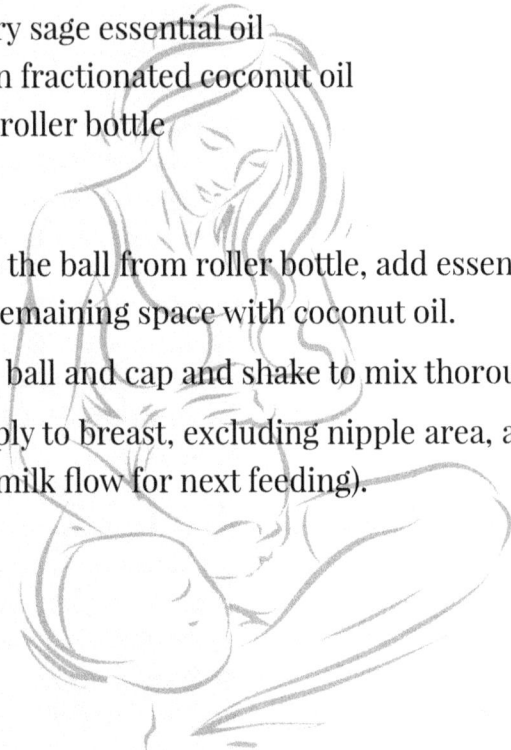

## *Milk Supply Roll-On*

**What You Will Need:**

4 drops geranium essential oil
2 drops fennel essential oil
1 drop rose essential oil
1 tablespoon jojoba oil
10 ml glass roller bottle

**What To Do:**

1. Remove the ball from the roller bottle and add essential oils.

2. Fill the remaining space with a carrier oil.

3. Replace ball and cap. Shake to blend.

**To Use:** Roll over the breasts between feedings. Be sure to wash the area before breastfeeding.

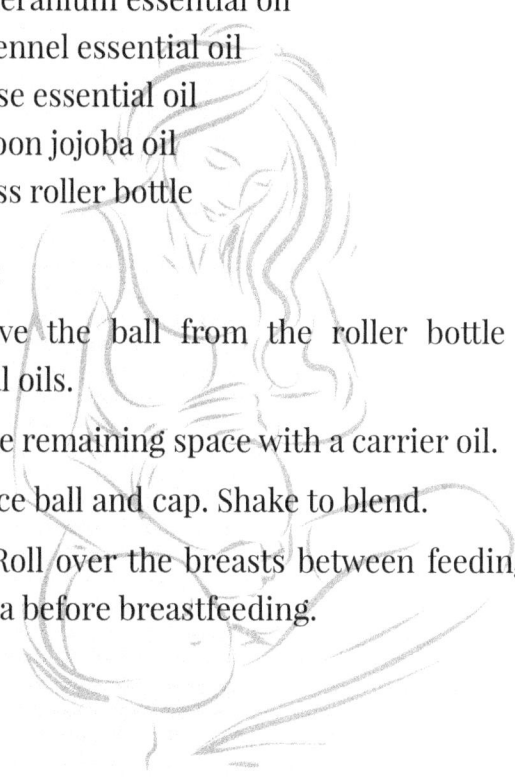

# Postpartum Depression

Due to all of the new responsibilities of having a baby on top of all of the crazy hormonal changes during the postpartum period, postpartum depression is a concern we really have to take into account. Symptoms includes sadness, changes in sleeping and eating patterns, low energy, anxiety, and irritability. Typically, the condition develops within 4 to 6 weeks after giving birth, but it can sometimes take several months to appear. It is not known why PPD occurs. However, depression is not a sign that you do not love your new arrival, as some mothers fear. It is a psychological disorder that can be effectively treated with the help of support groups, counseling, and essential oils.

Using essential oils aromatically can help support a new mom experiencing postpartum depression. Essential oils that can help include bergamot, clary sage, frankincense, geranium, grapefruit, mandarin, neroli, patchouli, rose, tangerine, vetiver, and ylang ylang.

## PPD Massage Oil

**What You Will Need:**

> 6 drops clary sage essential oil
> 6 drops geranium essential oil
> 6 drops mandarin essential oil
> 6 drops grapefruit essential oil
> 6 drops patchouli essential oil
> 6 drops ylang ylang essential oil
> 2 ounces grapeseed oil
> 2-ounce bottle

**What To Do:**

1. In a bottle, add essential oils and carrier oil.

2. Replace cap and shake to blend.

**To Use:** Massage into your entire body, or take it to your masseuse and ask her to use it once a week. You can also use at home as a neck massage oil daily or massage into the bottoms of your feet at night before bedtime.

## *Postpartum Depression Bath Soak*

**What You Will Need:**

>   3 drops geranium essential oil
>   3 drops frankincense essential oil
>   2 drops lavender essential oil
>   2 drops neroli essential oil
>   dead sea salts or himalayan salts
>   2-ounce tub or container

**What To Do:**

In a container, add salts and essential oils.

Stir to mix well. Store until ready for use.

**To Use:** Add bath salts to a running bath. Stir and agitate the water to dissolve. Soak in the tub for 20 minutes.

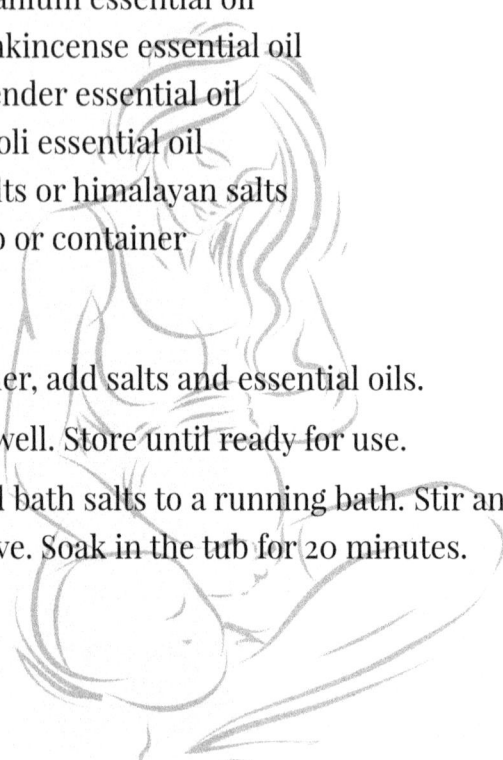

# Infant Care with Essential Oils

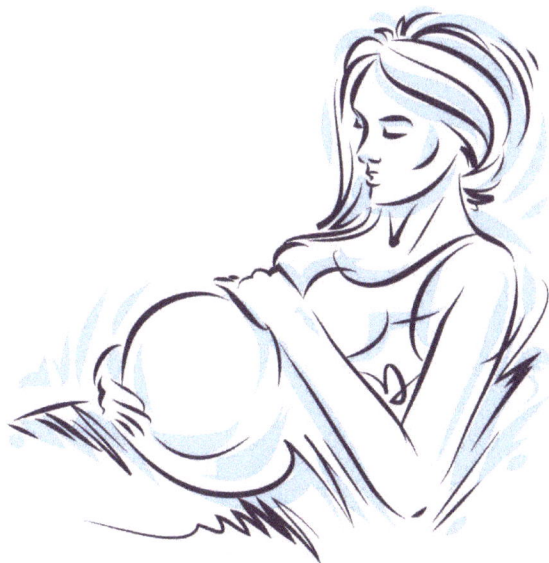

baby's body and brain develop at an astounding rate in the first year of life. Your tiny newborn quickly morphs into a curious, active little human eager to explore the world. Before you know it, your baby is a toddler.

An important safety note: use the gentlest essential oils available with the lowest rate possible. It is recommended to use .5% dilution or less for any infant care. Little bodies are sensitive and fragile, and we don't want to overwhelm their little system. Whenever possible, use hydrosols instead of essential oils as they are much gentler in action.

Besides using essential oils sparingly on babies, you need to ensure the essential oils used are safe for babies. Be careful not to diffuse essential oils around your little one. Also, make sure you wash off any essential oils off that have been applied to your breast prior to nursing the baby.

Essential oils safe for babies include German chamomile, Roman chamomile, lavender, mandarin, orange, tangerine, and tea tree (after six months).

## Umbilical Care

It's important to keep the umbilical cord clean and dry until the stump falls off. However, if it begins to turn red or starts to ooze, using a hydrosol can be helpful. Hydrosols that are recommended include Roman chamomile, lavender, and tea tree.

Hydrosols can be used safely on the baby after baths to help them calm down and relax, to soothe skin issues, and to treat cradle cap. Just a spritz of the hydrosol is all you need to use.

# Infant Massage

Infants enjoy light massage. Lightly running fingers over the baby's back, face and legs can help the baby relax and fall asleep peacefully. A highly diluted Roman chamomile or lavender essential oil blend (diluted with a carrier oil) can be very relaxing for the little one.

# Diaper Rash

If the baby's bottom becomes irritated, it could be caused by different reasons. It could be an allergic reaction to the chemicals in the diapers, wipes, or creams used. Or, it could be a fungal infection, eczema, or psoriasis. Essential oils that possess antibacterial, antifungal, and skin-nourishing properties are recommended—lavender, chamomile, tea tree, rosalina, palmarosa, frankincense, geranium, orange, neroli, petitgrain are a few of the oils that can be used to soothe and heal diaper rash.

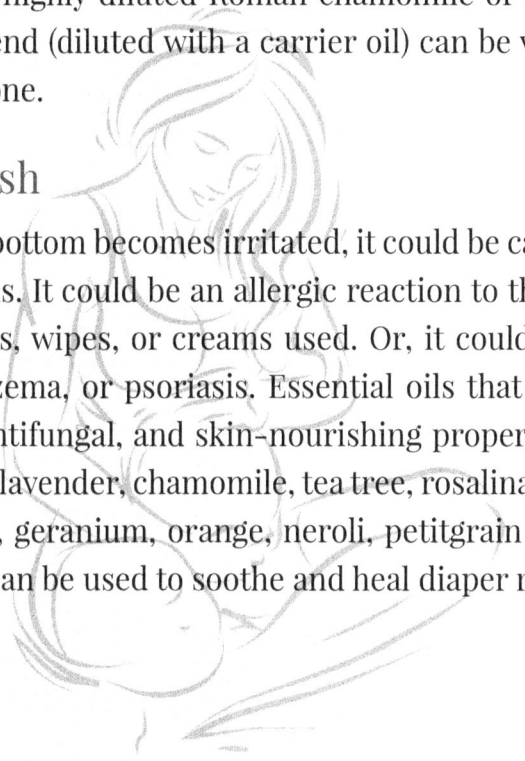

## Diaper Rash Cream

**What You Will Need:**

empty jar
double boiler
stir rod
6 drops tea tree essential oil
6 drops lavender essential oil
¼ cup shea butter
¼ cup coconut oil
1 tablespoon beeswax
1 tablespoon bentonite clay

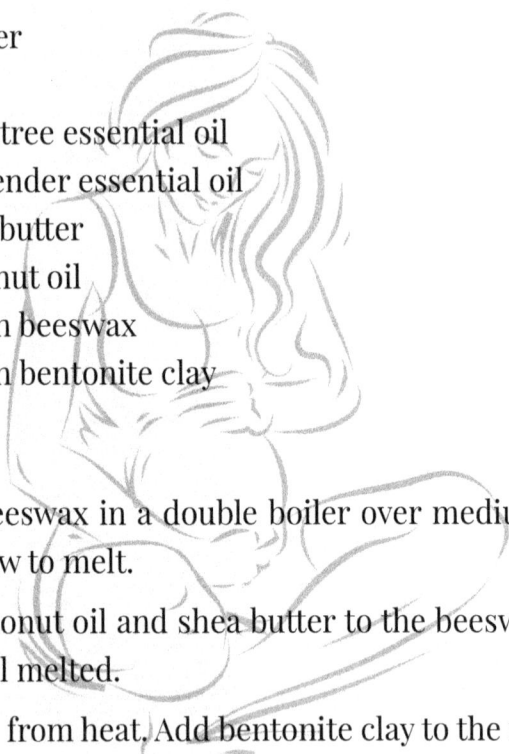

**What To Do:**

1. Place beeswax in a double boiler over medium-low heat and allow to melt.

2. Add coconut oil and shea butter to the beeswax mixture; stir until melted.

3. Remove from heat. Add bentonite clay to the mixture, stir well and allow to cool for 1-2 minutes.

4. Add the essential oils and stir to mix thoroughly.

5. Pour the mixture into a clean, glass jar. Place the lid on your jar and allow to cool completely before use.

**To Use:** Apply a thin coating over the baby's bottom at diaper changes.

# Abdominal Discomfort

Most babies will certainly at one time or another experience intestinal discomfort or tummy troubles. You can either gently massage your baby's abdomen in clockwise motion with the following mixture of essential oils and carrier oil or run a bath as described below.

An effective blend for such an occasion includes:

- 1 drop roman chamomile
- 1 drop sweet orange
- 2 teaspoons of carrier oil or baby bubble bath solution

Mix the essential oils in a carrier oil or bubble bath and add to running bath water before bathing your baby.

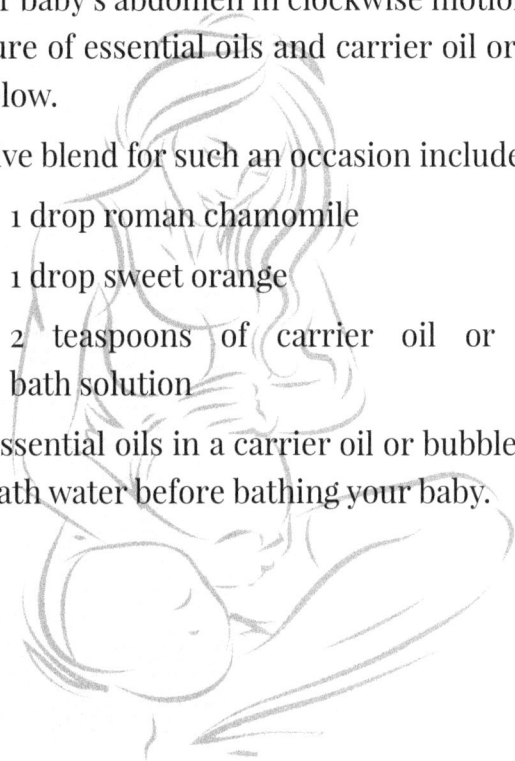

# Colds and Flu

For times where you're either trying to protect your baby from a cold that's circulating or are helping them fight one off, use these simple blends to keep the air fresh while also shortening the duration of a cold.

*Baby Flu Buster Blend*

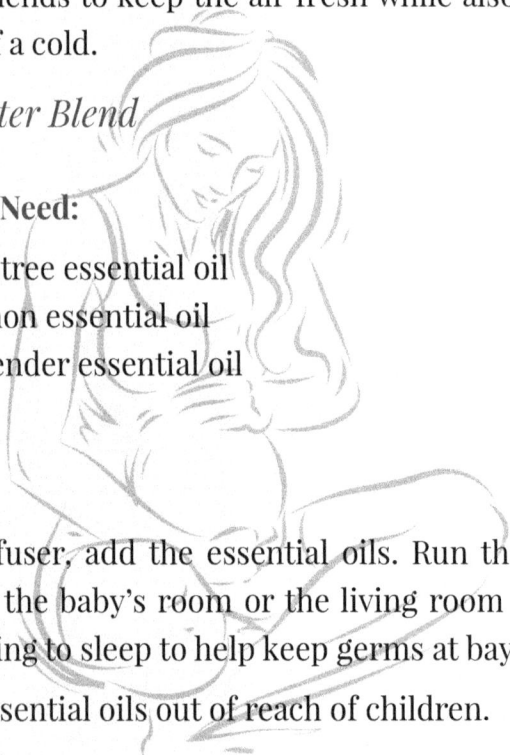

**What You Will Need:**

    2 drops tea tree essential oil
    2 drops lemon essential oil
    2 drops lavender essential oil
    diffuser

**What To Do:**

1. In a diffuser, add the essential oils. Run the diffuser ½ hour in the baby's room or the living room prior to the baby going to sleep to help keep germs at bay.

2. Store essential oils out of reach of children.

## *Baby Immuno-Boost Oil*

**What You Will Need:**

1 drop tea tree, lemon, or lavender essential oil
2 tablespoons coconut oil

**What To Do:**

1. In a small glass bowl, add one drop of essential oil to the carrier oil.

2. Stir to blend well.

**To Use:** Take a small amount of the mixture into your hand and massage the chest, back, and abdomen 2-3 times daily.

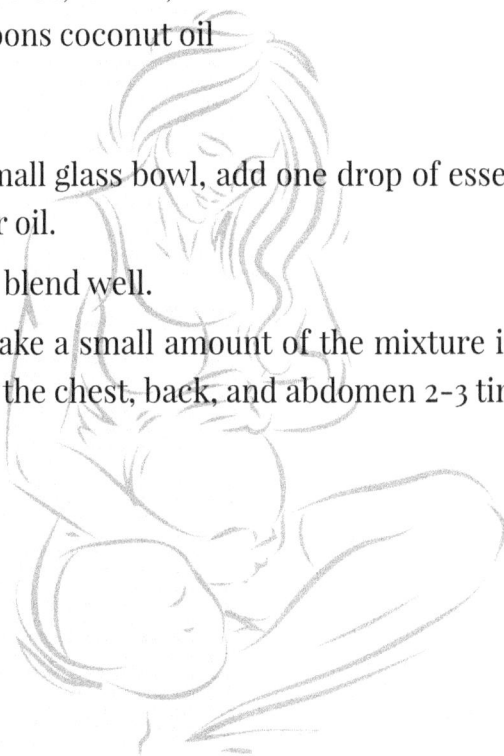

# Other Infant Care Tips:

## *Colic*

If your healthy baby frequently fusses and cries over long periods of time, he or she may have colic. To bring comfort to the baby, add one drop of Roman chamomile to one teaspoon of carrier oil and gently rub the abdomen, back, and feet.

## *Cradle Cap*

If your baby develops crusty white or yellow scales on the scalp, wash with a gentle shampoo and removes scales with a soft brush. Then, add one drop of geranium to one teaspoon of carrier oil. Gently massage into the scalp.

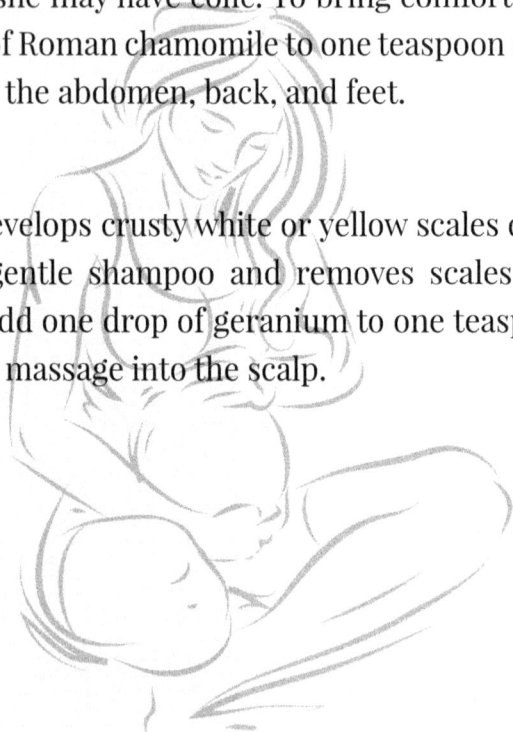

# Research on Essential Oils and Pregnancy

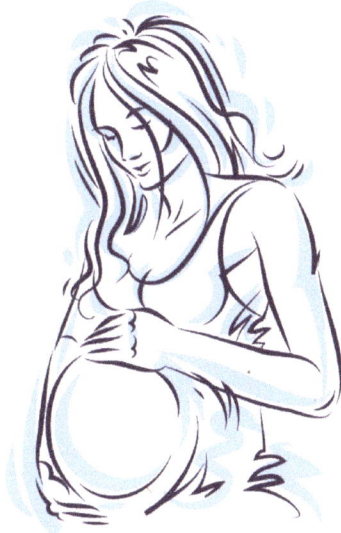

The following are some scientific studies that have been done on essential oil use during pregnancy and labor, as well as links to the full studies.

## Research Abstract on Nausea, Anxiety, and Pain

Clinical aromatherapy is the use of essential oils for clinical outcomes that are measurable, for example, nausea, anxiety, or pain. Essential oils are highly complex mixtures distilled from aromatic plants. They can be useful during pregnancy, labor, delivery, and postpartum. Essential oils can be applied in several different ways and are simple and pleasant to use. Essential oils are lipophilic. This paper will give an overview of published research relevant to maternal health, followed by examples of how aromatherapy is currently being used in a large maternity hospital, and give suggestions to encourage further integration."

**Link to Full Study:**

https://www.researchgate.net/publication/268522996_Clinical_Aromatherapy_for_Pregnancy_Labor_and_Postpartum

# Research Abstract on Lavender for Postpartum

"Lavender oil aromatherapy starting in the first hours of the postpartum period resulted in better physical and mood status compared to the non-aromatic group."

**Link to Full Study:**

https://www.ncbi.nlm.nih.gov/pmc/articles/PMC5439291/

# Research Abstract on Use of Aromatherapy in Childbirth

"This article discusses findings from a large evaluative study on the use of aromatherapy in childbirth (Burns et al., 1999). The sample involved 8058 mothers and took place in the delivery suite of a busy teaching unit. A primary objective was to examine whether aromatherapy could facilitate maternal coping mechanisms during labor by improving mothers' sense of wellbeing, reducing anxiety and fear, and influencing the perception of pain. Mothers consistently rated the administration of aromatherapy positively. Aromatherapy was found to be an inexpensive choice for mothers. Only 100 mothers reported minor side-effects associated with essential oil administration. This study provides a valuable insight into the potential for the use of aromatherapy in midwifery practice."

**Link to Full Study:**

https://www.researchgate.net/publication/272450347_Aromatherapy_in_childbirth_An_effective_approach_to_care

# Research Abstract on Essential Oils for Labor Pain

Aromatherapy refers to the medicinal or therapeutic use of essential oils absorbed through the skin or olfactory system. Recent literature has examined the effectiveness of aromatherapy in treating pain. *Methods.* 12 studies examining the use of aromatherapy for pain management were identified through an electronic database search. A meta-analysis was performed to determine the effects of aromatherapy on pain. *Results.* There is a significant positive effect of aromatherapy (compared to placebo or treatments as usual controls) in reducing pain reported on a visual analog scale (SMD = $-1.18$, 95% CI: $-1.33$, $-1.03$; $p< 0.0001$). Secondary analyses found that aromatherapy is more consistent for treating nociceptive (SMD = $-1.57$, 95% CI: $-1.76$, $-1.39$, $p < 0.0001$) and acute pain (SMD = $-1.58$, 95% CI: $-1.75$, $-1.40$, $p < 0.0001$) than inflammatory (SMD = $-0.53$, 95% CI: $-0.77$, $-0.29$, $p < 0.0001$) and chronic pain (SMD = $-0.22$, 95% CI: $-0.49$, $0.05$, $p = 0.001$), respectively. Based on the available research, aromatherapy is most effective in treating postoperative pain (SMD = $-1.79$, 95% CI: $-2.08$, $-1.51$, $p < 0.0001$) and obstetrical and gynecological pain (SMD = $-1.14$, 95% CI: $-2.10$, $-0.19$, $p < 0.0001$). *Conclusion.* The findings of this study indicate that aromatherapy can successfully treat pain when combined with conventional treatments."

**Link to Full Study:**

https://www.ncbi.nlm.nih.gov/pmc/articles/PMC5192342/

# Resources

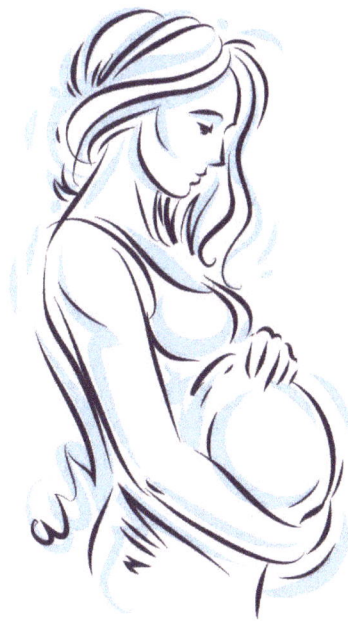

T he following pages are resources to help you in using essential oils safely during your pregnancy, labor, delivery, and postpartum care.

- Dilution Chart
- Quick Reference Condition Chart
- Therapeutic Properties Glossary

## Dilution Chart

|       | 5 ml | 10 ml | 15 ml | 20 ml | 25 ml | 30 ml | 50 ml | 100 ml |
|-------|------|-------|-------|-------|-------|-------|-------|--------|
| .5%   | .75  | 1.5   | 2.25  | 3     | 3.75  | 4.5   | 7.5   | 15     |
| 1%    | 1.5  | 3     | 4.5   | 6     | 7.5   | 9     | 15    | 30     |
| 2%    | 3    | 6     | 9     | 12    | 15    | 18    | 30    | 60     |
| 3%    | 4.5  | 9     | 13.5  | 18    | 22.5  | 27    | 45    | 90     |
| 4%    | 6    | 12    | 18    | 24    | 30    | 36    | 60    | 120    |
| 5%    | 7.5  | 15    | 22.5  | 30    | 37.5  | 45    | 75    | 150    |

# Quick Reference Condition Chart

| CONDITION | ESSENTIAL OILS |
|---|---|
| **PREGNANCY** | |
| Abdominal Discomfort | Juniper, Benzoin, Lavender, Mandarin |
| Acne | Bergamot, Geranium, Lavender, Lemon, Lime, Mandarin, Neroli, Niaouli, Palmarosa, Petitgrain, Rose, Sandalwood, Tea Tree |
| Anxiety | Bergamot, Virginian Cedarwood, Roman Chamomile, Frankincense, Jasmine, Lavender, Lemon, Lime, Marjoram, Neroli, Palmarosa, Patchouli, Rose, Sandalwood, Vetiver, Ylang Ylang, Orange |
| Backache | Black Pepper, Eucalyptus, Ginger, Lavender, Lemon, Peppermint, Pine |
| Breast Tenderness | Black Pepper, Cypress, Frankincense, Helichrysum, Lavender, Geranium, German or Roman Chamomile, Marjoram, Rosalina, Ylang Ylang |

| CONDITION | ESSENTIAL OILS |
|---|---|
| Constipation | Black Pepper, Ginger, Orange, Peppermint, Pine, Rosemary |
| Depression | Bergamot, Roman Chamomile, Frankincense, Geranium, Jasmine, Lavender, Lemon, Mandarin, May Chang, Neroli, Peppermint, Pine, Rose, Sandalwood, Tangerine, Ylang Ylang |
| Dizziness | Frankincense, Peppermint, Pine |
| Edema and Swelling | Cypress, Geranium, Grapefruit, Juniper Berry, Mandarin, Orange, Rosemary, Tangerine |
| Fetal Positioning | Peppermint, Pine, Spearmint, Siberian Fir |
| Frequent Urination | Sweet Marjoram, Cypress |
| Group B Strep/ Bacterial Vaginosis | Lavender, Tea Tree |
| Headache | Eucalyptus, Roman Chamomile, Lavender, Lemon, Neroli, Peppermint |

| CONDITION | ESSENTIAL OILS |
|---|---|
| Heartburn | Black Pepper, Cajeput, German Chamomile, Roman Chamomile, Cypress, Eucalyptus, Ginger, Mandarin, Neroli, Peppermint, Petitgrain, Sandalwood, Spearmint |
| Hemorrhoids | Cypress, Frankincense, Geranium, Helichrysum, Lavender, Juniper Berry, Peppermint, Orange, Sandalwood |
| Insomnia | Bergamot, Roman Chamomile, Lavender, Lemon, Neroli, Petitgrain, Orange, Sandalwood, Vetiver |
| Leg Cramp | Bergamot, Roman Chamomile, Copaiba, Cypress, Geranium, Lavender, Peppermint |
| Charley Horse | Roman Chamomile, Copaiba, Cypress, Geranium, Lavender, Peppermint, Rosemary |
| Morning Sickness | Petitgrain, Orange, Mandarin |
| Nausea/Vomiting | Black Pepper, Cardamom, German Chamomile, Roman Chamomile, Ginger, Peppermint |

| CONDITION | ESSENTIAL OILS |
|---|---|
| Preeclampsia | Bergamot, Roman Chamomile, Frankincense, Geranium, Lavender, Lemon, Lime, Orange, Sandalwood |
| Fatigue | Geranium, Grapefruit, Lavender, Lemon, Orange, Peppermint |
| Flatulence | Black Pepper, Cardamom, Roman Chamomile, Cumin, Dill, Ginger, Lavender, Peppermint, Spearmint |
| PUPPS | German Chamomile, Roman Chamomile, Lavender, Helichrysum, Patchouli, Sandalwood |
| Round Ligament Pain | Black Pepper, Roman Chamomile, Lavender |
| Sciatica | Black Pepper, Cajeput, German Chamomile, Eucalyptus, Ginger, Lavender, Nutmeg, Peppermint |
| Stretch Marks | Frankincense, Geranium, Helichrysum, Lavender, Neroli, Rose, Roman Chamomile, Tangerine |
| Urinary Tract Infection | Cypress, Grapefruit, Lemon, Lime |

| CONDITION | ESSENTIAL OILS |
|---|---|
| Varicose Veins | Cypress, Geranium, Lemon, Orange, Sandalwood |
| Water Retention | Petitgrain, Geranium, Grapefruit, Fennel |
| Yeast Infection | Bergamot, German Chamomile, Lavender, Lemongrass, Tea Tree |

**LABOR & DELIVERY**

| | |
|---|---|
| Back Labor | Black Pepper, Ginger, Marjoram, Peppermint, Rosemary |
| Mastitis | Clary Sage, Geranium, Helichrysum, Lavender, Neroli, Rose |
| Blood Pressure | Bergamot, Clary Sage, Helichrysum, Lavender, Neroli, Rose |
| Contractions | Black Pepper, Clary Sage, Geranium, Jasmine, Marjoram, Neroli |
| Increasing Lactation | Clary Sage, Fennel, Geranium, Rose |
| Muscle Tension | Black Pepper, Cypress, Lavender, Marjoram, Peppermint |

| CONDITION | ESSENTIAL OILS |
| --- | --- |
| Perineal Care | Frankincense, Helichrysum, Lavender, Tea Tree |
| Labor Progression | Clary Sage, Fennel, Lavender, Jasmine, Neroli, Rose |
| Transition | Bergamot, Clary Sage, Grapefruit, Jasmine, Lemon, Lime, Mandarin, Orange, Patchouli, Rose, Rosemary, Spearmint |
| C-Section Wound Care | Frankincense, Helichrysum, Lavender, Tea Tree |
| Episiotomy Care | Frankincense, Helichrysum, Lavender, Tea Tree, Petitgrain |
| Exhaustion | Grapefruit, Bergamot, Orange, Lemon, Lime, Spearmint |

**MOMMY CARE**

| | |
| --- | --- |
| Cracked/Dry Nipples | Roman Chamomile, Geranium, Helichrysum, Lavender, Rose |
| Fatigue | Bergamot, Grapefruit, Lemon, Orange, Rosemary, Spearmint |
| Milk Production | Clary Sage, Fennel, Geranium |

| CONDITION | ESSENTIAL OILS |
|---|---|
| Postpartum Depression | Bergamot, Clary Sage, Frankincense, Geranium, Grapefruit, Mandarin, Neroli, Patchouli, Rose, Tangerine, Vetiver, Ylang Ylang |
| Sore Breasts | Roman Chamomile, Cypress, Geranium, Lavender |

**INFANT CARE**

| | |
|---|---|
| Umbilical Care | Hydrosols, Roman Chamomile, Lavender |
| Infant Massage | Hydrosols, Roman Chamomile, Lavender |
| Diaper Rash | Hydrosols, Lavender, Roman Chamomile, Tea Tree, Rosalina, Palmarosa, Frankincense, Geranium, Orange, Neroli, Petitgrain |

# Therapeutic Properties

When studying about each essential oil, you will want to be familiar with their therapeutic properties, understanding their action to determine which oils to avoid and which oils will be beneficial during pregnancy and postpartum and for infant care.

**Abortifacient** – induces premature expulsion of a fetus from the uterus.

**Analgesic** – relieves pain.

**Antibiotic** – inhibits the growth of bacteria and prevents it from spreading.

**Anticoagulant** – prevents the clotting of blood.

**Antiemetic** – reduces or alleviates nausea and vomiting.

**Antiphlogistic** – reduces inflammation and fever.

**Antiseptic** – inhibits or stops the growth of microorganisms.

**Antispasmodic** – prevents or stops spasms or cramps.

**Aperitif** – stimulates the appetite.

**Carminative** – moves gas from the stomach or intestines.

**Cordial** – stimulating.

**Demulcent** – soothes irritated mucous membranes and relieves pain and inflammation.

**Depressant** – eases nervousness.

**Digestive** – aids in the digestive process.

**Diuretic** – aids in toxin elimination; increases urination and helps rid the body of excess fluid.

**Emmenagogue** – regulate the body's hormonal flow in the female reproductive system.

**Galactagogue** – promotes breast milk production and secretion.

**Hemostatic** – slows down or stops bleeding.

**Laxative** – causes the bowels to empty themselves.

**Nervine –** calming to the nervous system; useful in stress and anxiety.

**Sedative** – calms the nerves with a tranquilizing effect upon the body, reducing stress or anxiety.

**Soporific** – promotes deep sleep.

**Vulnerary** – aids in healing or treating wounds and helps to prevent tissue degeneration.

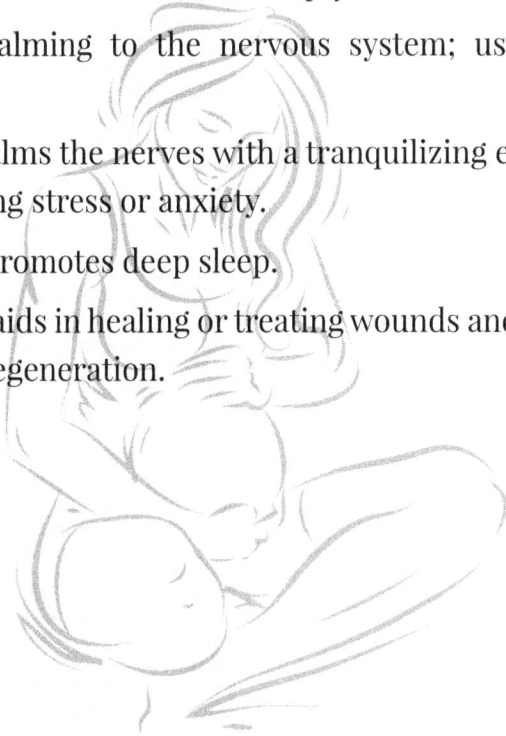

# Other Books by Rebecca Park Totilo

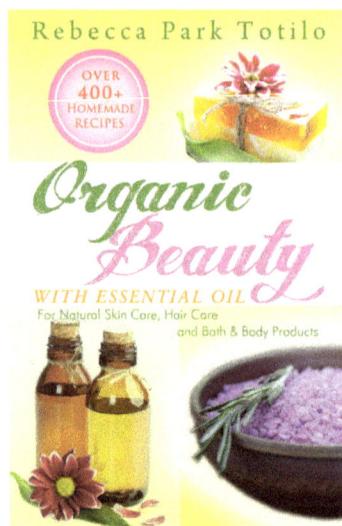

*Organic Beauty With Essential Oil: Over 400+ Homemade Recipes for Natural Skin Care, Hair Care and Bath & Body Products*

Sweep aside all those harmful chemically-based cosmetics and make your own organic bath and body products at home with the magic of potent essential oils! In this book, you'll find a luxurious array of over 400 Eco-friendly recipes that call for breathtaking fragrances and soothing, rich organic ingredients satisfying you head to toe. Included you'll find helpful can have the confidence knowing which essential oil to use and how much when creating your own body scrub, lip butter, or lotion bar! Discover how easy it is to make bath treats like fragrant shower gels, dreamy bubble baths, luscious creams and lotions, deep cleansing masks and facials for literally pennies using essential oils and ingredients from your kitchen.

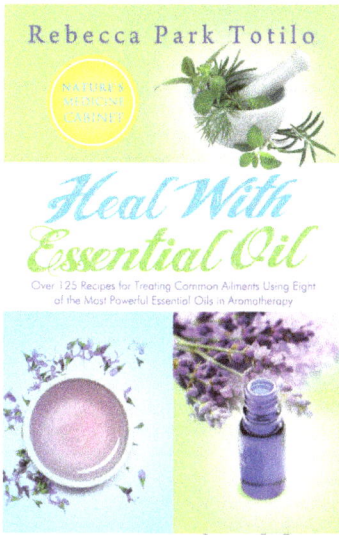

### *Heal With Essential Oil: Nature's Medicine Cabinet*

Using essential oils drawn from nature's own medicine cabinet of flowers, trees, seeds and roots, man can tap into God's healing power to heal oneself from almost any pain. Find relief from many conditions and rejuvenate the body. With over 125 recipes, this practical guide will walk you through in the most easy-to-understand form how to treat common ailments with your essential oils for everyday living. Filled with practical advice on therapeutic blending of oils and safety, a directory of the most effective oils for common ailments and easy to follow remedies chart, and prescriptive blends for aches, pains and sicknesses.

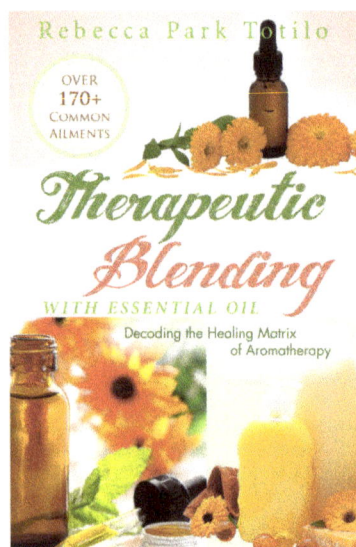

### Therapeutic Blending With Essential Oil: Decoding the Healing Matrix of Aromatherapy

Therapeutic Blending With Essential Oil unlocks the healing power of essential oils and guides you through the intricate matrix of aromatherapy, with a compilation of over 170 common ailments. Discover how to properly formulate a blend for any physical or emotional symptom with easy to follow customizable recipes. Now, you can make your own massage oils, hand and body lotions, bath gels, compresses, salve ointments, smelling salts, nasal inhalers and more. This exhaustive guide takes all the guesswork out of blending oils from how many drops to include in a blend, to measuring thick oils, to how often to apply it for acute or chronic conditions. It also shows you how to create a single blend for multiple conditions. Even if you run out of oil for a favorite recipe, this book shows you how to substitute it with another oil.

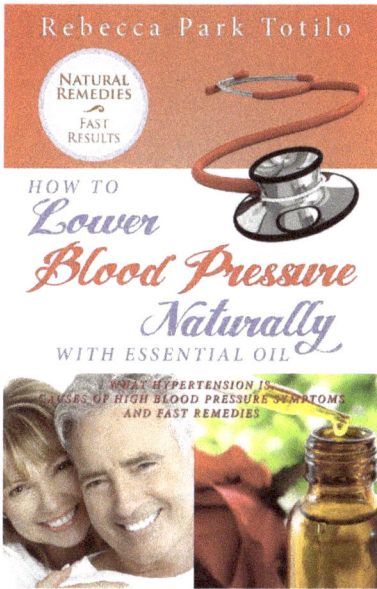

*How To Lower Blood Pressure Naturally With Essential Oil: What Hypertension Is, Causes of High Pressure Symptoms and Fast Remedies*

One out of three adults have it, and another one-third don't realize it. Oftentimes, it goes undetected for years. Even those who take multiple medications for it still don't have it under control. It's no secret -- high blood pressure is rampant in America. High blood pressure, or hypertension, has become a household term. Between balancing meds and monitoring diets though, are the true causes -- and best treatments -- hidden in the shadows? In How to Lower Blood Pressure Naturally With Essential Oil, Rebecca Park Totilo sheds light on what high blood pressure is, the causes and symptoms of high blood pressure, and which essential oils regulate blood pressure and how to use essential oils as a natural, alternative method.

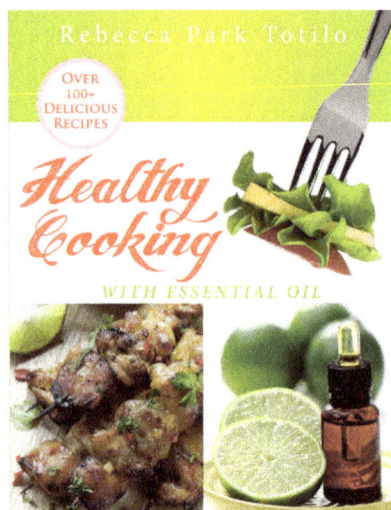

### Healthy Cooking with Essential Oil

Imagine transforming an everyday dish into something extraordinary using only a drop or two of essential oil can enliven everything from soups, salads, to main dishes and desserts. Boasting flavor and fragrance, these intense essences can turn a dull, boring meal into something appetizing and delicious. Essential oils are fun, easy-to use and beneficial, compared to the traditional stale, dried herbs and spices found in most pantries today. Healthy food should never be thought of as mere fuel for the body, it should be enjoyed as a multi-sensory experience that brings therapeutic value as well as nourishment. For years we have limited the use of essential oils to scented candles and soaps, in the belief that they were unsafe to consume (and some are!). However, more people are realizing the value of using pure essential oils to enhance their diet. In Healthy Cooking With Essential Oil, you will learn how cooking with essential oils can open up a wealth of creative opportunities in the kitchen.

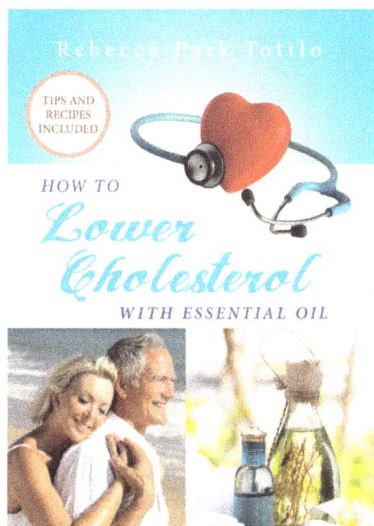

### *How to Lower Cholesterol with Essential Oil*

Take healthy steps now to control high cholesterol and its risk factors with essential oils. People with high cholesterol have twice the risk for heart disease according to the Center for Disease Control and Prevention. What's worse, most folks aren't even aware that they have atherosclerosis until they have a heart attack or stroke. Lowering your cholesterol and triglycerides with essential oils may slow, reduce, or even stop the buildup of dangerous plaque in your arteries causing blockage of blood flow which could result in a heart attack or stroke. In this indispensable guide, author Rebecca Park Totilo presents scientific research supporting the efficacy of certain essential oils for lowering cholesterol, an extensive essential oil and carrier oil directory, natural treatments with recipes, along with easy-to-follow methods of use via inhalation, topically, and ingestion.